The Treatment of External Diseases with Acupuncture and Moxibustion

The Treatment of External Diseases with Acupuncture and Moxibustion

Yan Cui-lan
Zhu Yun-long

BLUE POPPY PRESS
BOULDER, CO

Published by:

Blue Poppy Press
1775 Linden Ave. Boulder, CO 80304
(303) 447-8372

First Edition January, 1997

ISBN 0-936185-80-5
Library of Congress #96-80188

Copyright © Blue Poppy Press

All rights reserved. No part of this book may be reproduced, stored in a retrieval system, or transcribed in any form, by any means electronic, mechanical, photocopy, recording, or other means, or translated into any other language without prior written permission of the publisher.

The information in this book is given in good faith. However, the translators and the publishers cannot be held responsible for any error or omission. Nor can they be held in any way responsible for treatment given on the basis of information contained in this book. The publishers make this information available to English readers for scholarly and research purposes only.

The publishers do not advocate nor endorse self-medication by laypersons. Chinese medicine is a professional medicine. Laypersons interested in availing themselves of the treatments described in this book should seek out a qualified professional practitioner of Chinese medicine.

COMP Designation: Original work using a standard translational terminology

Printed at Bookcrafters in Chelsea, MI

10, 9, 8, 7, 6, 5, 4, 3, 2, 1

Editor's Preface

In the early 1980s when acupuncture and Chinese medicine were relatively new and undeveloped in the West, I wrote a book called *Tieh Ta Ke: Traditional Chinese Traumatology & First Aid.* However, after selling well for several years, we let this book go out of print as our knowledge of Chinese medicine made it evident that this book was far from adequate. Ever since, I have wanted to publish a translation of a good Chinese *wai ke* or external medicine text, traumatology or *shang ke* being a subdivision of *wai ke*. Therefore, I was happy to hear that one of our Blue Poppy Press translators, Yang Shou-zhong, had an acupuncture and moxibustion colleague who was a specialist in *wai ke,* and, what's more, this colleague wanted to publish her book on the acupuncture and moxibustion treatment of *wai ke* diseases through Blue Poppy Press.

Therefore, we are pleased to offer this acumoxa therapy text on the treatment of *wai ke* diseases to Western practitioners of Chinese medicine worldwide. It is one more step in Blue Poppy Press's goal of providing basic textbooks on all the specialties of Chinese medicine. In this book, the reader will find a wealth of information on the Chinese medical disease causes and mechanisms, pattern discrimination, and acupuncture-moxibustion treatment of dozens of dermatological, traumatological, orthopedic, and other external diseases as categorized by Chinese medicine. This is an area of Chinese medicine which is not well known by Westerners, and the fact that the author is primarily an acupuncturist, as are the majority of Western practitioners of Chinese medicine, makes this book especially appropriate for Western readers.

Western readers should note that the author has arranged this book by traditional Chinese disease categories. These are followed in the chapter titles by modern Western disease names where appropriate. As a member of the Council of Oriental Medical Publishers (COMP), Blue Poppy's standard for the identification of acupoints is the World Health Organization's Standard Acupuncture Point Nomenclature with the following deviations: First, instead of channel abbreviation and point number followed by Pinyin name in parentheses, we present the Pinyin name first with the channel abbreviation and point number following in parentheses. Secondly, we have separated each Pinyin word. New Jersey is not written Newjersey in English. Similarly, we believe *He Gu,* meaning Union Valley should not be run on, just as one would not write Union valley in English. Third, as for channel and vessel abbreviations we have changed LU to Lu, ST to St, SP to Sp, HT to Ht, BL to Bl, KI to Ki, PC to Per, TE to TB, and LV to Liv. And fourth, for extra-channel points, our standard is Nigel Wiseman's *Glossary of Chinese Medical Terms and Acupuncture Points*, Paradigm Publications, Brookline, MA, 1990.

Bob Flaws
Boulder, CO

Foreword

Two years ago I visited the United States as the guest of Blue Poppy Press. One of the things that left a deep impression on me is the rapid growth in acceptance of acupuncture in that country. One episode in particular stands out in my memory. One day, my friend, Charles Chace, a well-known acupuncturist, translator, and teacher of Chinese medicine in his own right, took me along to see one of his patients. The patient was a woman who had been involved in a traffic accident and had a bad multiple fracture. When she learned that I also taught and practiced Chinese medicine, the woman expressed to me her great satisfaction of the effects of acupuncture on her rehabilitation. Until then, I had thought that Americans knew no more of acupuncture than its pain-relieving effect and that such a case would have been hospitalized and treated by a modern Western medical orthopedist. From this encounter, it is apparent that Western acupuncturists are facing a larger diversity of cases and more serious cases than many Chinese practitioners think.

Chinese medicine is roughly divided into *nei ke* or internal medicine and *wai ke* or external medicine. In the last several years, a number of books have been published in English on *nei ke*. In general, *nei ke* focuses on diseases of the viscera and bowels, at least as conceived by Chinese medicine. However, there is little that has yet been translated into English on *wai ke*, and, as the above case illustrates, Western practitioners are treating what in China would be considered *wai ke* patients. The category of *wai ke* includes diseases of the skin, the muscles and flesh, and the sinews and bones. As such, *wai ke* encompasses several specialties of Western medicine, including orthopedics, rheumatology, traumatology, neurology, and even dermatology. Therefore, this book should be a welcome addition to the clinical libraries of Western practitioners of acupuncture and Chinese medicine.

Dr. Yan Cui-lan, the principal author of this book, is a skilled and experienced acupuncturist with high attainment in many branches of Chinese medicine. I have known her for a number of years. After graduation from a medical institute, she began her career as an acupuncturist in the teaching hospital of the Northern China Coal Mines Medical College in Tangshan, Hebei, where I also work. From then till now, she has been in practice for over 20 years. Her name first came to my attention one day when I was checking the list of borrowers of books from the college library. To my surprise, nearly every book on Chinese medicine and acumoxa therapy in which I was interested contained the name Yan Cui-lan on its list of borrowers. Thus I was impressed by this person's wide reading. Having become aware of her name, I soon noticed that she was also a prolific writer, for I now recognized that her name appeared in this or that medical journal as well. Although I was not yet personally acquainted with this lady, I could imagine and respected her diligence. By chance it occurred that, one year later, the two of us were assigned together to teach acupuncture and moxibustion lessons to foreign students. This assignment has given me the chance to get to know Yan Cui-lan both as a colleague and friend.

In the past, many Chinese medical authors have included the word "heart" in the title of their books, for instance the *Dan Xi Zhi Fa Xin Yao (The Heart & Essence of Dan-xi's Treatment Methods)*. This word heart in Chinese signals the reader that such a book contains the personal experience of the author and is not just a compilation of other peoples' thoughts, words, and experiences. Although this book, *The Treatment of External Diseases with Acupuncture & Moxibustion*, does not contain the word heart in its title, this book really is Dr.Yan's heart book. In this book, Dr. Yan shares the fruits of her own extensive clinical experience with other acupuncturists. Although a scholar in her own right and though she often uses quotes from various classics and old Chinese medical texts to substantiate and clarify her statements, nonetheless, this book is not just the stale textbook repetition of the standard party line on this subject. Rather, it is one clinician's record of a lifetime of experience in the acupuncture and moxibustion treatment of a wide range of external diseases.

In addition, this book bears another unique distinction. It is being published first in English through Blue Poppy Press Inc. before it appears in Chinese. Dr. Yan wrote this book with the assistance of Zhu Yun-long. It was then translated into English by Li Jian-yong using a standard translational terminology as it appears in Nigel Wiseman's *English-Chinese Chinese-English Dictionary of Chinese Medicine*, Hunan Science & Technology Press, Changsha, 1995. Readers should note that some key terms have been retranslated in this dictionary from how they appear in Nigel Wiseman's *Glossary of Chinese Medical Terms and Acupuncture Points,* Paradigm Publications, Brookline, MA, 1990.

Yang Shou-zhong
Tangshan, Hebei

Table of Contents

Editor's Preface v
Foreword vii

Book One: Introduction

1 A Short History of Chinese External Medicine Vis à Vis Acumoxatherapy 1
2 Disease Causes & Disease Mechanisms 5
3 The Essentials of Pattern Discrimination 9
4 A General Discussion of Treatment 15
5 Needling Methods 19
6 Methods of Moxibustion 25
7 Cupping 29
8 A Guide to Point Selection 31

Book Two: Dermatoses & Infectious Sores

1 Introduction 35
2 Nodulations (Furuncles) 41
3 Welling Abscesses (Carbuncles) 45
4 Flat Abscesses (Acute Cellulitis) 49
5 Headless Flat Abscesses (Pyogenic Osteomyelitis & Arthritis) 53
6 Clove Sores (Pyogenic Infection or Malign Boils) 55
7 Cinnabar Toxins (Erysipelas) 59
8 Scrofulous Lumps 61
9 Bloated Cheeks (Mumps) 63
10 Sloughing Flat Abscesses (Thromboangitis Obliterans) 67
11 Breast Welling Abscesses (Acute Mastitis) 71
12 Shank Sore (Varicosity Syndrome) 77
13 Steeping Sap Sore (Eczema) 81
14 Addictive Papules (Urticaria) 83
15 Snake Cinnabar (Herpes Zoster) 87
16 Oxhide Lichen (Neurodermatitis) 91
17 Warts 93
18 Chicken's Eyes (Corns) 99
19 Bedsores 101
20 Drinker's Nose (Acne Rosacea) 103

21 Frozen Sore (Frostbite & Hypothermia) 107
22 Pricking Powder (Acne Vulgaris) 111
23 White Patch Wind (Vitiligo) 113
24 White Sores (Psoriasis) 115
25 Wet Foot Qi (Athlete's Foot) 119
26 Wind Glossy Scalp (Alopecia Areata) 121

Book Three: Animal Bites

1 Bee & Wasp Sting 125
2 Poisonous Snake Bite 127
3 Rabid Dog Bite (Rabies) 131

Book Four: Orthopedics & Traumatology

1 Fracture 135
2 Wrenching of the Low Back (Acute Lumbar Sprain) 141
3 Forked Qi (Upper Back Sprain) 143
4 Sinew Binding (Ganglion Cyst) 143
5 Heel Pain 145
6 Tail Bone Pain 147
7 Damaged Sinews (Wrist & Ankle Sprain) 149
8 Flaccid Body (Traumatic Paraplegia) 153

Book Five: Impediment

1 Exposed Shoulder Wind (Periarthritis of the Shoulder) 159
2 Taxed Elbow (Tennis Elbow) 163
3 Jumping Round Wind (Sciatica) 165
4 Skin Impediment (Cutaneous Neuritis) (1) 167
5 Skin Impediment (Localized & Systemic Scleroderma) (2) 169
6 Sinew Impediment (Myotenositis Musculi Supraspinati) (1) 175
7 Sinew Impediment (Rhomboideus Strain) (2) 177
8 Neck & Shoulder Pain (Cervical Spondylosis) 179
9 Articular Wind (Rheumatic Arthritis) 183
10 Deformation Impediment (Rheumatoid Arthritis) 189
11 Thigh Wind (Piriformis Syndrome) 191
12 Chest & Rib-Side Pain (Costal Chondritis) 193
13 Mandibular Pain (Temporomandibular Joint Syndrome) 195
14 Crick in the Neck (Torticollis) 197

21 Frozen Sore (Frostbite & Hypothermia) 109
22 Pricking Powder (Acne Vulgaris) 113
23 White Patch Wind (Vitiligo) 115
24 White Sores (Psoriasis) 117
25 Wet Foot Qi (Athlete's Foot) 121
26 Wind Glossy Scalp (Alopecia Areata) 123

Book Three: Animal Bites

1 Bee & Wasp Sting 127
2 Poisonous Snake Bite 129
3 Rabid Dog Bite (Rabies) 133

Book Four: Orthopedics & Traumatology

1 Fracture 137
2 Wrenching of the Low Back (Acute Lumbar Sprain) 143
3 Forked Qi (Upper Back Sprain) 145
4 Sinew Binding (Ganglion Cyst) 145
5 Heel Pain 147
6 Tail Bone Pain 151
7 Damaged Sinews (Wrist & Ankle Sprain) 153
8 Flaccid Body (Traumatic Paraplegia) 157

Book Five: Impediment

1 Exposed Shoulder Wind (Periarthritis of the Shoulder) 163
2 Taxed Elbow (Tennis Elbow) 167
3 Jumping Round Wind (Sciatica) 169
4 Skin Impediment (Cutaneous Neuritis) (1) 171
5 Skin Impediment (Localized & Systemic Scleroderma) (2) 173
6 Sinew Impediment (Myotenositis Musculi Supraspinati) (1) 179
7 Sinew Impediment (Rhomboideus Strain) (2) 181
8 Neck & Shoulder Pain (Cervical Spondylosis) 183
9 Articular Wind (Rheumatic Arthritis) 187
10 Deformation Impediment (Rheumatoid Arthritis) 193
11 Thigh Wind (Piriformis Syndrome) 195
12 Chest & Rib-Side Pain (Costal Chondritis) 197
13 Mandibular Pain (Temporomandibular Joint Syndrome) 199
14 Crick in the Neck (Torticollis) 201

Book Six: Anal Diseases

1 Prolapse of the Rectum ... 203
2 Hemorrhoids ... 207
3 Splitting of the Anus (Anal Fissure) ... 209
4 Sitting Wind (Perianal Eczema) ... 211

Book Seven: Tumors

1 Goiter ... 215
2 Tofu-dregs Tumor (Sebaceous Cyst) ... 219
3 Mammary Node (Mammary Fibroadenoma) (1) ... 221
4 Mammary Node (Fibrocystic Breast Condition) (2) ... 225

Book Eight: Postoperative & Miscellaneous Troubles

1 Helping Heal the Cut ... 229
2 Postoperative Nausea, Retching & Vomiting ... 231
3 Postoperative Abdominal Distention & Constipation ... 233
4 Hiccough ... 235
5 Urinary Block (Urinary Retention) ... 239
6 External Kidney Welling Abscess (Acute Orchitis) ... 241
7 Intestinal Welling Abscess (Appendicitis) ... 243

Index ... 247

Table of Contents

Editor's Preface v
Foreword vii

Book One: Introduction

1 A Short History of Chinese External Medicine Vis à Vis Acumoxatherapy 1
2 Disease Causes & Disease Mechanisms 5
3 The Essentials of Pattern Discrimination 9
4 A General Discussion of Treatment 15
5 Needling Methods 19
6 Methods of Moxibustion 25
7 Cupping 29
8 A Guide to Point Selection 31

Book Two: Dermatoses & Infectious Sores

1 Introduction 35
2 Nodulations (Furuncles) 41
3 Welling Abscesses (Carbuncles) 47
4 Flat Abscesses (Acute Cellulitis) 51
5 Headless Flat Abscesses (Pyogenic Osteomyelitis & Arthritis) 55
6 Clove Sores (Pyogenic Infection or Malign Boils) 57
7 Cinnabar Toxins (Erysipelas) 61
8 Scrofulous Lumps 63
9 Bloated Cheeks (Mumps) 65
10 Sloughing Flat Abscesses (Thromboangitis Obliterans) 69
11 Breast Welling Abscesses (Acute Mastitis) 73
12 Shank Sore (Varicosity Syndrome) 79
13 Seeping Sap Sore (Eczema) 83
14 Addictive Papules (Urticaria) 85
15 Snake Cinnabar (Herpes Zoster) 89
16 Oxhide Lichen (Neurodermatitis) 93
17 Warts 95
18 Chicken's Eyes (Corns) 101
19 Bedsores 103
20 Drinker's Nose (Acne Rosacea) 105

Book Six: Anal Diseases

1 Prolapse of the Rectum ... 199
2 Hemorrhoids ... 203
3 Splitting of the Anus (Anal Fissure) ... 205
4 Sitting Wind (Perianal Eczema) ... 207

Book Seven: Tumors

1 Goiter ... 211
2 Bean-dregs Tumor (Sebaceous Cyst) ... 215
3 Mammary Node (Mammary Fibroadenoma) (1) ... 217
4 Mammary Node (Fibrocystic Breast Condition) (2) ... 221

Book Eight: Postoperative & Miscellaneous Troubles

1 Helping Heal the Cut ... 225
2 Postoperative Nausea, Retching & Vomiting ... 227
3 Postoperative Abdominal Distention & Constipation ... 229
4 Hiccough ... 231
5 Urinary Block (Urinary Retention) ... 235
6 External Kidney Welling Abscess (Acute Orchitis) ... 237
7 Intestinal Welling Abscess (Appendicitis) ... 239

Index ... 243

Book One: Introduction

1
A Short History of Chinese External Medicine *vis à vis* Acumoxatherapy

The treatment of various external traumas and sores has been a part of Chinese medicine right from its start. In the *Ling Shu (The Spiritual Pivot),* there is a whole chapter devoted to sores titled "Welling Abscesses & Flat Abscesses" (Ch. 80), and in quite a number of other chapters, external problems are also discussed at some length. The chapters, "Migratory *Bi"* (Ch. 27) and "The Treatise on Pain" (Ch. 53), are examples. Although it is *The Spiritual Pivot* which mainly deals with acupuncture and moxibustion, the *Su Wen (Simple Questions)* is also not lacking in discussions on the acupuncture and moxibustion treatment of external troubles. In these two works many specific acupuncture and moxibustion treatments are recorded concerning such external traumas as welling abscesses (acute infammatory lesion), flat abscesses (obstinate chronic lesion), rat's scrofula (tuberculous lymphadenitis), and heel marrow illness (osteomyelitis). It is a well known fact that the basic acupuncture and moxibustion treatment principles in external medicine were already established in these two classics more than 2,000 years ago. In a discussion of the treatment of axillary welling abscesses, the *Simple Questions* instructs:

> Puncture five points on the foot *shao yang*. If heat refuses to abate, puncture three points on the hand heart governor and three points each on the hand *tai yin* network vessels and the meeting places of the bones.

The routes of the three channels mentioned in this instruction all run across the axilla. That is to say, the approach to treating external troubles in these two classics is based on the theory of the channels and network vessels, and this principle is the cornerstone of Chinese medicine and acupuncture to this day.

When China entered the era of the Jin down through the Six (Succeeding) Dynasties (265-581 CE), the most noticeable achievement in the realm of external medicine was the publication of the *Zhou Hou Bei Ji Fang (Emergency Formulas [to Keep] Behind the Elbow)* by Ge Hong (281-341 CE) in which more than 20 different moxibustion methods are recorded for external diseases. In addition, Ge Hong is credited with the invention of a number of new moxibustion methods, such as moxaing over garlic or salt, all of which have been preserved to this day as effective moxibustion options. Another event meriting attention in this period was the publication of the *Liu Juan Zi Gui Yi Fang (Master Liu Juan's Ghost left Formulas)*. This is possibly the first work in China specializing in external medicine. It is a tremendously rich treasure house of acupuncture and moxibustion in this sphere. In it, there are no few efficacious acupuncture and moxibustion treatment methods. One of them is the so-called encircling moxibustion method which can be illustrated by the following instructions contained in this book:

> First moxa (the center of the sore) with 200-300 cones. Then moxa its sides with 100-200 cones at four points for a small-sized sore, six points for a medium-sized one, and 8 points for a large-sized one...

Another important work from this period is the *Xiao Pin Fang (A Concise Formulary Book, Concise Book* hereinafter) by Chen Yan-zhi, who advocated the combined use of fire needles, long needles, and medication.

The Sui and its succeeding dynasty, the Tang, ushered in the most prosperous era in Chinese history. With the flourishing of the nation in every aspect of its life, medicine enjoyed a very favorable period of development. Great medical works were published in large numbers. The *Zhu Bing Yuan Hou Lun (Treatise on the Origins & Symptoms of the Various Diseases, The Origins* hereinafter) by Chao Yuan-fang, the *Qian Jin Fang (Formulas [Worth A] Thousand [Pieces of] Gold, Thousand Pieces of Gold* hereinafter) by Sun Si-miao, and the *Wai Tai Mi Yao (Secret Essentials of the External Platform, External Platform* hereinafter) by Wang Tao are the most eminent among the many valuable medical works published in this period. In these products of the great minds of Chinese medicine of this time, there is a predilection for moxibustion for the treatment of external diseases such as welling abscesses and flat abscesses, and, as moxibustion became more important, moxibustion methods became more varied. It was during this time that medicated mugwort cones or cones of mugwort mixed with some other appropriate specific medicinals were introduced. This considerably enhanced the efficacy of moxatherapy. However, this does not mean that during this period practitioners neglected acupuncture. In the *Qian Jin Yi Fang (The Supplement to the Formulas [Worth] a Thousand [Pieces of] Gold, Supplement* hereinafter), for example, we can read an instruction for treating hemorrhoids:

> *Chang Qiang* (GV 1) ... is the ruling point for the five types of hemorrhoids... Insert the needle to a depth of 3 *cun* while the patient is made to lie prostrate... Moxibustion is also good, but not as (good as) needling.

The years from the Song down through the Yuan dynasty (960-1368 CE) saw the maturity of acumoxatherapy in China. This was marked by the historical event of casting the bronze model of the acupoints and channels. At the time, external medicine developed greatly not only in extent but in depth as its own medical specialty. Acupuncturists by then had a wealth of sophisticated means for identifying various kinds of external and internal injuries. In the *Tai Ping Sheng Hui Fang (The Imperial Grace Formulary of the Tai Ping [Era])* by Wang Huai-yin *et al.,* there was a whole chapter devoted to welling and flat abscesses in which a detailed discussion of the pathology, disease mechanisms, clinical diagnosis, and specific acupuncture and moxibustion treatment of such lesions were given. According to this book, one can simply determine whether or not there are tender places at the *mu* points of the viscera and bowels in order to detect internal welling abscesses.

> If there is a dull pain at the (lung) alarm point, Zhong Fu (Lu 1), there is lung welling abscess. This can also be verified if the flesh there is a little raised.

In addition, a whole group of works specializing in acupuncture and moxibustion for external problems came into the world at this time, such as the *Wai Ke Jiu Fa Lun Cui Xin Shu (A New Book of Pithy Treatises on Moxibustion Methods in External Medicine)* by Xu Meng-fu, the *Yong Ju Jiu Fa (Moxibustion Methods for Welling & Flat Abscesses)* by Liu He-shu, and the *Qi Zhu Ma Jiu Fa (Riding the Bamboo Horse Moxibustion Method)*. The four great masters of the Jin-Yuan period-Liu Wan-su, Zhang Zi-he, Li Dong-yuan, and Zhu Dan-xi-each made some precious contribution to the culmination of this discipline. Their doctrines are all based on the *Nei Jing (Inner Classic)* and, as a group, they developed a practical and more comprehensive analysis of various external injuries based on channel and network vessel theory. It follows that they advanced the principle of point selection in accordance with the (affected) channels. Before this time, point selection for external lesions was mainly based on the use of local points. Liu Wan-su said, "For all species of sores indicating acupuncture and moxibustion, it is necessary to determine which channel and network vessel is affected and, subsequently, to determine the amount of qi and blood there and the distance (of the lesion to the center)." According to him, if sores break out on the back, one should select among the five transporting points of the *tai yang*, i.e., the well, spring, stream, river, and sea points. If they develop on the face, one should choose among the five transporting points of the *yang ming*. If they appear on the lateral side of the head, one should treat among the five transporting points of the *shao yang*.

If the previous ages were years of exploration, sowing the seeds and cultivating the plants, the Ming and Qing dynasties (1368-1911 CE) were the time of harvesting. As to this period, one may be disappointed if one expects to find marked progress in theory. Rather, people during this time occupied themselves with collecting the experiences and insights of their predecessors, and, in their clinical practice, they distinguished themselves by their ability to synthesize the application of all relevant previous theories. The many works titled *A Great Collection* or something similar (*i.e. Da Quan, Da Cheng,* etc.) prove this proclivity towards collection, standardization, and synthesis in the medical scholarship this age.

2
Disease Causes & Disease Mechanisms

What is so-called external medicine in terms of Chinese medicine? In Chinese medicine, there seems to be no clear-cut demarcation between internal and external medicine. Roughly speaking, external medicine is the study of diseases which are mainly located in the superficial tissues, *i.e.*, the skin, the muscles and flesh, and the sinews and bone. For the treatment of external troubles, Chinese traditionally have resorted primarily to the application of pastes, steaming and fumigation, simple surgical operations, or acupuncture and moxibustion rather than the oral administration of internal medicine, although the latter may be included as an adjunctive treatment. Sometimes, however, cases like appendicitis, where an internal organ is involved, may also be included within the scope of Chinese external medicine. However, this latter approach may be the product of the influence of modern Western medicine. In the past, the equivalent of external medicine (*wai ke*) was called the specialty in sores (*yang ke*). This term had a narrower definition than modern *wai ke*. For instance, in the old classics, appendicitis appeared by the name of intestinal welling abscess and was discussed under the category of internal medicine. Therefore, we can see that, nowadays, external medicine embraces those diseases which would otherwise be treated by surgery in modern Western medicine. Hence, *wai ke* is often translated functionally as surgery in the English language literature.

Disease causes

In Chinese medicine, there is something called three causes theory, and this theory is well-suited to external medicine. This theory was first advanced in the work, the *San Yin Ji Yi Bing Zheng Fang Lun (The Treatise on Diseases, Their Symptoms & Formulas According to the Uniform Theory of Three Causes)* by Chen Wu-ze (1131-1189 CE). According to Chen, all disease causes can be divided into external, internal, and neither external nor internal causes. Based on this book, we can identify the causes of external diseases as follows.

1. External attack by the six environmental excesses

Unlike the internal organs, the superficial tissues and particularly the skin are exposed with little or no protection. Therefore, their diseases are more often due to environmental factors, such as untimely changes in the weather, a damp living environment, or overly cold or hot weather. When an external evil invades the body, it first settles in the skin and muscles. If it is cold, it will congeal the qi and blood, impeding their flow. If it is heat, it may make the defensive slack, forcing open the interstices. In either case, a sore or a pain may develop.

2. Traumatic accidents

Accidental injuries from falls, boiling water, fire, chemicals, and physical contact with irritants or abrasion or insect or snake bites may cause disorder of the qi and blood resulting in blood stasis. Thus the channels and network vessels are blocked and, therefore, various lesions arise. (Traumatic accidents fall under Chen's category of neither external nor internal causes of disease.)

3. Internal Damage

Internal damage is also often responsible for external troubles. Such internal damage may result from viscera and bowel disharmony in turn caused by constant worry and anxiety, anger and vexation, protracted stress, or sudden violent disturbance of the spirit. These emotional disturbances force the ethereal and corporeal souls to soar, leaving the viscera and bowels vacuous and empty or making them depressed. When the ethereal and corporeal souls are not in their proper position, external evils have a chance to invade and wreak havoc. Excessive sexual intercourse is also a culprit in external problems which should not be overlooked. It may deplete the kidney essence, upsetting the penetrating and controlling (formally called penetrating and conception) vessels[1], and causing disharmony of the qi and blood. Moreover, overtaxation may damage the spleen, the central earth, and, as a result, there will appear insufficiency of the source of generation and transformation. The kidneys govern the earleer heaven or prenatal qi, while the spleen is in control of the latter heaven[2] or postnatal qi. Thus they play a crucial role in keeping the body fit and strong. If either of these two viscera becomes disordered, this may express itself in the exterior.

In his *Yi Men Fa Lu (Rules & Laws Within the Gate of Medicine),* Yu Jia-yan (1585-1664 CE) said:

> Every type of sore has some causes... As regards internal disease causes, mellow wine and rich flavors produce heat toxins, while immoderate depression and fury engender fire toxins...

---

[1] Wiseman gives thoroughfare vessel for chong mai replacing his previous penetrating vessel. The translator feels this is one of the few instances where Wisemna's revised terms are worse than his original ones. Therefore, we have retained penetrating.

[2] Wiseman gives later haven for *hou tian*. We use latter. We regard this as only a stylistic difference which we prefer for the sound.

This quote reminds us of the importance of an appropriate diet and healthy eating habits. Overeating greasy, hot, and acrid flavors may damage the spleen qi, causing damp heat toxins to accumulate. In that case, damp heat toxins may erode the skin and flesh, causing sores.

Disease mechanisms

Next we come to disease mechanisms. After evils invade the body, the righteous qi will rise up against them. The outcome of the battle between evil and righteous qi decides the progression of the disease. In other words, the possibility and the speed of recovery are dependent upon the balance and interaction between these two. In this regard, particular consideration should be given to the conditions of the viscera and bowels and the channels and network vessels.

1. Qi & blood

Qi and blood circulate together around the body without a break to maintain normal life activities. If the qi and blood are affected, stagnation or congelation of them may arise. In that case, they are held up in a certain part, blocked possibly in the muscles, possibly in the sinews, possibly in the bones, giving rise to such as sores. The *Inner Classic* says, "When the circulation of the constructive qi is at a stop and there is counterflow in the interstices of the flesh, welling abscess swelling develops there." This instruction tells us that qi and blood stasis marks the onset of such problems as sores.

The *Ling Shu (The Spiritual Pivot)* has a passage giving a more detailed account of the course of development of sores in the chapter "The Treatise on Welling & Flat Abscesses" which says:

> The constructive and defensive are thus confined (to some place) in the channel vessel. In consequence, the blood is congested, its circulation at a stop. When the constructive qi is at a stop, the defensive is also blocked. It is congested and arrested; therefore, heat is generated. This heat may become fulminant and endless. When it prevails, the flesh putrefies. Putrefied flesh produces pus.

The *Wai Ke Mi Lu (Secret Records of External Medicine)* published in 1694 says:

> So long as the qi and blood are effulgent, external evils cannot affect (the body). But when the qi and blood are debilitated, the internal righteous will no longer be able to resist them.

This terse saying is pregnant with meaning. Effulgent qi and blood are a strong defense. Should evils by chance invade and produce swellings and sores, these swellings and sores will easily break, and it will not be difficult for new flesh and muscle to grow. If the qi is vacuous, it will have difficulty in filling up and breaking the swellings and sores, for vacuous yang qi now has no easy access to the surface of the body. If there is a shortage of blood, since blood is not sufficient to provide nourishment for the muscles, it is not easy for new muscle, i.e., flesh, to grow after the swellings and sores are open. In general, swelling preceding pain is due to damage of the qi, while pain preceding swelling is due to damage of the blood. A hard swelling is due to binding of the qi and blood. Redness of the affected flesh shows abundance of qi and blood, while gray or whitish flesh demonstrates debilitation of qi and blood. In sum, the qi and blood presuppose the course as well as the generation of swellings and sores.

2. Viscera & bowels

Although external troubles are usually located in the exterior, they often concern the internal organs. The *Wai Ke Qi Xuan (Enlightening the Subtleties of External Medcine)* by Shen Dou-huan published in 1604 CE says:

> All types of sores arise from disharmony of the five viscera and congestion of the six bowels. This disharmony and congestion leads to blockage of the channels and vessels, and, as a result, sores are produced. For example, either depression and binding of the liver qi or damp heat of the spleen may cause sores. This is what is meant by the saying, "What exists in the interior will manifest itself in the exterior."

On the other hand, pathologic changes in the exterior may affect or advance into the interior, resulting in pathologic changes in the viscera and bowels. Take a clove sore on the face for example. This species of sore engenders effulgent heat toxins. These toxins may then take advantage of insufficiency of the qi and blood to diffuse, attacking inward the viscera and bowels and developing into what is called evil fire assaulting the heart (septicema). When toxic qi strikes the heart, various mental disorders, like clouded spirit and raving, will arise. These evil toxins may offend the lungs. In that case, coughing of blood and chest pain will appear. When an external trouble is complicated by a visceral or bowel disorder, the prognosis is usually bad.

3. Channels & network vessels

The channels and network vessels originate in the viscera and bowels, running throughout the whole body, reaching every part of the body, the skin, the blood vessels, the sinews, the bones, and the flesh. They connect the various organs and the various tissues into an integrated whole. They are the highways and roads of the righteous qi, blood, and fluids, and for evils as well. Therefore, pathogens of any kind, either endogenous or exogenous, will invariably affect the channels and their network vessels, causing blockage and congestion of them somewhere. On the other hand, when the channels and their network vessels are involved, some innocent parts, the qi and blood in particular, will inevitably be the next victims. The qi and blood stagnate and become obstructed, and hence swellings and sores arise. There is a famous maxim in the *Wai Ke Jing Yao (The Essence & Essentials of External Medcine)* by Xue Ji (1486-1558 CE) that welling and flat abscesses are originally the product of fire toxins arising from blocked channels and network vessels and the congelation of qi and blood. In connection with swellings and sores, it is through the channels and network vessels that the evils or toxins are transmitted inward to attack the viscera and bowels or outward from the viscera and bowel to the exterior of the body.

3
The Essentials of Pattern Discrimination

External medicine follows basically the same principles as internal medicine in regard to pattern discrimination. In treating external troubles, it is no less significant to go by the theories of the viscera and bowels, the channels and network vessels, the qi and blood, and the fluids and humors. The four examinations and the eight principles also hold good in external medicine as well.

Local signs & symptoms

However, since local pathologic changes are conspicuous in external troubles, local signs and symptoms should be given more attention in diagnosis and treatment. Different types of external disease display different signs and symptoms, and hence different pathogens can be tracked down. Effulgent heat produces putrified flesh and copious exudation and manifests as localized redness and burning pain in the exterior. Swelling reveals blockage of the channels and network vessels, while pain is due to qi and blood stasis. As a disease cause, dampness is identified by fixed pain, as in rheumatism, and much exudation, as in sores.

What's more, the kind of pathogen has something to do with the location of the external trouble. In general, sores developing in the upper part of body, including the head and face, the neck, and the upper limbs, are usually due to wind heat, for wind heat is inclined to ascend. Sores seen in the middle part of the body, including the chest, upper back, and abdomen, are often a result of qi or fire depression, for qi and fire originate in the center. As for sores in the lower part of the body, cold dampness is responsible in most cases, for dampness tends to descend.

As to the examination of local lesions, it is necessary to discuss this at some more length. The commonly and often simultaneously seen main local manifestations include redness, swelling, heat, pain, and suppuration. Through a synthesized study of these, one may be able to deepen their knowledge about the lesions in question.

1. Redness & heat

Redness and heat are the result of fire and heat. Fire is classified into vacuity fire and repletion fire, and, in terms of its location, there is a distinction between the qi and blood divisions or aspects. In relation to their origin, fire may be a consequence of invading external toxins, may be transmuted from protracted depression, or may be generated from excessive vacuity. The first kind is repletion fire. This typically gives the affected area a bright red color and a burning heat. The second kind is vacuity fire which is characterized by a faint red color and slight or no heat of the affected area. If fire involves the qi division, there is heat but no redness. Acute lymphadenitis is an example of this. Fire affecting the blood division is characterized by both redness and heat. Aggression of external fire toxins, as in clove sores and furuncles, produces redness and heat at the very onset. Protracted depression transmuting into fire is also characterized by redness and heat, but it progresses slowly. Tubercular lymphadenitis is a case of fire transmuted from protracted despression. In connection with fire toxins generated internally, redness and heat usually appear in the initial stage, preceded and accompanied by disorder of the viscera and bowels.

2. Pain & swelling

Pain and swelling are reactions to the blockage and stagnation of the qi and blood of the channels and network vessels. There is the saying, "Pain is none other than a reflection of blockage." The *Yi Xue Ru Men (Entering the Gate of Medicine, Entering the Gate* hereinafter) by Li Yan published in 1575 CE says:

> Pain preceding swelling is ascribed to damage of the blood. Swelling preceding pain is ascribed to damage of the qi. Simultaneous attacking of swelling and pain is ascribed to damaged qi and blood.

In the case of swelling preceding pain, the problem usually lies shallowly in the skin and flesh, while pain preceding swelling reveals that the trouble lies deep in the sinews and bones.

3. Pus

Pus is transformed and generated from qi and blood. *Entering the Gate* says, "Effulgent heat putrefies the flesh and putrefied flesh turns into pus." *The Inner Classic* says:

> Heat is the producer of pus. However, without dampness, it cannot erode the muscles and flesh to turn them into pus.

From the above classical statements, it is clear that the cause of pus is damp heat. To determine whether pus has developed or not, one can place their fingers over the swelling. If they can perceive a rippling sensation, there is pus. Otherwise, there is no pus. Another method of detecting pus is to study the color of the lesion. If there is a dark shade under the skin, there is pus. If no dark shade can be discerned, there is no pus yet.

Study of the characteristics of pus may yield valuable information. If the pus is yellow, thick, and has no strange odor, there is still abundant qi and blood left. If the pus is yellowish white, the righteous qi is not shown to be short. If the pus looks filthy and thin and smells rancid, then the qi and blood are debilitated. If the pus is thin and rancid and the overlying skin of the lesion is encircled by a black color, there are long-accumulated toxins having damaged the sinews and putrefied the bone. The prognosis in that case is unfavorable.

When a sore is open, giving forth pus, the condition may turn for the better if generalized systoms are abating or disappearing. If there is no marked improvement seen in the general condition, the trouble is progressing.

4. Itching

Itching is an expression of inhibited circulation of the qi and blood within the skin and flesh. Generally speaking, if there is only slight heat, there is itching. If there is abundant heat, there is pain.

If itching happens in the initial stage of a disease, it is the product of the contention between wind dampness and wind heat. If it happens in the course of treatment, it shows restoration of the qi and blood. It is noteworthy, however, that improper treatment may also provoke itching.

5. Aching

Aching, a dull vexing pain, is indication of inhibited flow of qi and blood in the sinews and bones. It is due to the three evils: wind, cold, and dampness. If wind is the predominant factor, the aching is migratory or episodic. If cold prevails, the aching is fixed and continuous. If dampness is the overwhelming factor, the aching is accompanied by a sensation of distention.

Generalized signs & symptoms

While we are observing the local symptoms, we should also make an equally careful study of the generalized signs and symptoms which are the second, yet no less important indeces in diagnosis.

In many cases, external diseases are complicated or accompanied by generalized systoms which differ in category and degree of their severity. These include cold shivering, fever, clouded head, headache, generalized pain and aching, no desire for food, constipation, short voidings of dark-colored, scanty urine, and, in severe cases, vexation and agitation, clouded spirit, raving, rapid, surging pulse, yellow, coarse tongue fur with a crimson tongue body, etc. Generalized signs and symptoms are direct expressions of the general condition of the body- the state of yin and yang, the viscera and bowels, and the qi and blood. In general, fulminant generalized systoms indicate a vigorous struggle put up by the righteous qi or rampant invading evil qi. On the other hand, less fulminant generalized reactions do not necessarily show that the problem is not serious. On the contrary, very often the problem may be critical. This then shows that the righteous qi is too weak to put up an effective resistance to the invading evils. This is most often seen in those cases where enduring disharmony of the viscera and bowels is the origin of the disease.

Since many kinds of external troubles are closely related to the internal viscera and bowels, one has to determine which is the priority in the treatment-the local lesion or the viscera and bowels. To reach a correct conclusion, it is vital to be clear about the relationship between the local signs and symptoms and the generalized ones. Suppose a skin lesion is localized and very severe, while there are only slight generalized systems. It may be justifiable to design a therapy specific for the local problem without the need to pay much attention to the viscera and bowels, the qi and blood, etc. If, on the contrary, we face a case of enduring flat abscess, a deep lesion into the flesh, which is accompanied by no fulminant generalized signs and symptoms but a white facial complexion, diminished qi, and a weak pulse, then one cannot achieve successful treatment unless one gives priority to supplementation of the qi and blood in general. The clinical experience of many outstanding Chinese physicians tells us that, as a safe policy, one had better always remind oneself against the fallacy of focusing the treatment merely on the local problem to the neglect of the general condition. Otherwise the treatment is often bound to be a failure. Furthermore, not only should we establish the priority of the local lesion over the general condition or vice versa, but we have to identify the nature of the disease.

Yin and yang are the head-ropes of the eight principles. Therefore it is of paramount importance to determine whether the trouble is a yin or yang pattern. Only then can one devise a correct treatment plan. The *Yang Yi Da Quan (The Great Collection for External Medicine Specialists)* by Gu Shi-cheng published in 1760 CE says:

> When examining and treating sores of any category, it is necessary to have a clear idea of yin and yang. Yin and yang are the head-ropes of the *dao* of medicine. When yin and yang are correctly identified, how can the treatment be wrong? Complex though the medical *dao* may be, it can be boiled down to just two words-yin and yang.

Cases of pronounced local and generalized systems, swift advancing, and hyperactivity are all ascribed to yang. As far as local manifestations are concerned, a yang pattern is characterized of sudden onset, rapid progression, affects only the shallow depth, and is accompanied by redness of the skin, burning heat, protruding localized swelling, acute pain, and thick pus. The generalized manifestations of a yang pattern include fever and chills, thirst, no desire for food, constipation, and short voidings of dark-colored, scanty urine. When the swelling opens, the above signs and symptoms gradually disappear. Sores of the yang pattern are easy to open, easy to disperse, easy to close, and hence easy to treat. In most cases, their prognosis is favorable.

If there are no marked local or generalized systems after evils have invaded, this shows that the righteous qi is weak and vacuous, and that the pattern is of a yin nature. The yin pattern progresses slowly and persists over a long time. It starts deep in the sinews or bones. The overlying skin takes on a dark purple or normal color with slight or no heat. The affected skin and flesh is sunken, and the swelling is diffuse rather than localized. There is no pain or only a slight, dull pain. The pus issuing from the lesion is thin, possibly mixed with fibrous materials. Although, in the initial stage, there are few, if any, ostensible generalized manifestations, in the advanced stage, tidal fever, spontaneous sweating, night sweats, red cheeks, or chalky white facial complexion may appear. When the swelling opens, the above manifestations may become more apparent. The yin pattern is difficult to disperse, difficult to open, and difficult to close. Its prognosis is bad.

4
A General Discussion of Treatment

Like other therapies in Chinese medicine, acupuncture and moxibustion in external medicine are based on a holistic view of the body in turn based on the collection of information about a given case through the four examinations. After the pattern is identified, one can design a treatment plan, deciding on whether to use needling, moxibustion, both together or also medication. As previously said, in many cases, the troubles are rooted in the interior. Therefore, the treatment plan often includes a combination of expulsion from within and external treatment. What is meant by expulsion from within and external treatment?

1. External treatment

External treatment is short-hand for treating the local and *a shi* points, aiming at directly and specifically affecting the local lesion for the purpose of stopping pain and promoting the maturation of pus for example. This is oftener than not a vital part of the treatment plan. The reason for this is easy to see. Take sores for example. They are usually localized and there must be a great binding of evil qi or accumulation of toxins in the local area. Unless serious efforts are made to directly disperse this binding or these toxins, the sores cannot be healed.

2. Explusion from within

Expulsion from within means not only draining the evils but supplementing the righteous. It takes the general condition of the body as its target. In other words, it is an effort to drive out the evils through regulating the viscera and bowels, harmonizing the qi and blood, and balancing yin and yang. Although expulsion from within may seem to act only indirectly on the superficial disease focus, it is very important nonetheless.

The human body is in constant communication with and under the constant influence of the outer macrocosm. When it is affected by unfavorable environmental factors, unfavorable changes in the interior of the body will occur which never fail to give some external somatic expression. On the other hand, since the body is an organic whole, a microcosm in its own right, every part is closely related to all the other parts. Therefore, unless it is an incised wound or injury from a fall, when facing external disease, one should *always* try to probe into the state of the viscera and bowels, the qi and blood, and the channels and network vessels in order to reveal the internal pathological changes before one can find a way to manage the problem. In fact, even when treating a cut, one should take into consideration the internal state of the viscera, determining whether yin and yang are in balance and whether the qi, blood, or both are excess or insufficient. In modern terms, one should always bear in mind the holistic point of view. In his *Wai Ke Zheng Zong (Orthodox Gathering of External Medicine, Orthodox Gathering* hereinafter), the famous physician, Chen Shi-gong (1555-1636 CE), said:

> An internal illness may not be expressed in the exterior, but external illnesses invariably have their roots in the interior...Therefore a superficial ailment may be practically (speaking) an incurable disease of the *gao huang*.

The *gao huang* is believed to lie in the innermost part of the body and a *gao huang* disease is hence a critical, life-threatening, and insidious condition.

This point of view is best summarized in a quote from *The Inner Classic* which states that, when the righteous qi is replenished, "Wind and rain, cold and heat are unable to make one vacuous because mere evils cannot do injury to people."

A common saying carries the same implication: "Evil qi brings damage to people, but it is abnomality that results in affection." Abnomality here means disorder in the interior which, in turn, refers to imbalance between yin and yang, excess or insufficiency of the viscera and bowels, disharmony of the qi and blood, etc. In other words, as long as the righteous qi keeps to the interior, no evil can do anything to the body or, though it is capable of causing some trouble, the righteous qi may get rid of it in time. Therefore, to prevent injury from external evils, one should try to keep their righteous qi effulgent by means of, among others, balancing work and rest and maintaining a cheerful frame of mind.

In order to directly affect the local lesion, as said previously, one should select local and *a shi* points. To supplement the center and boost the qi as a general approach, such points as *Qi Hai* (CV 6), *Guan Yuan* (CV 4), and *San Li* (St 36), for example, are necessary besides other appropriate important points on the related channels. Thus the combination of local and distant points must be synergistic, in order to accelerate the recovery of external troubles like wounds and sores.

In order to affect both the local and general conditions, the practitioner must also be proficient in needle and moxibustion hand technqiues, and this issue will be discussed in the next few chapters.

The actions of acupuncture & moxibustion

Knowing about the actions of acupuncture and moxibustion is closely related to the concepts of expulsion from within and external treatment. As far as external medicine is concerned, first of all, acupuncture and moxibustion may accomplish dispersion. Dispersion is the prevention of the development of toxins before sores and swellings have become fulminant. In his *Wai Ke Shu Yao (Pivotal Essentials of External Medicine)* published in 1571 CE, Xue Ji said:

> In the treatment of sores, it is essential to try to disperse them before they become mature. If they are treated early enough, even though they may otherwise be a major problem, they will have to vanish before they have taken shape.

The Orthodox Gathering says:

> Before sores have developed for seven days, they are not mature in shape or threatening, while the righteous qi is not made weak. Whether they are a pattern of yin or yang, cold or heat, vacuity or repletion, it is necessary to perform moxibustion. Thus, in mild cases, the toxic qi will be dispersed by fire, while in severe cases, depressed toxins will be drawn out. Then the interior and exterior will be both unblocked.

The above quotations tell us the significance of opportune dispersion.

It seems that moxibustion is a satisfactory means of dispersing toxins. In fact, it really is because it is able to warm the channels and scatter cold, dispel wind and eliminate dampness, disperse phlegm and scatter nodulation. However, needling is also capable of dispersing toxins, for it can resolve the exterior and free the interior, course the liver and resolve depression, free the flow of the channels and quicken the network vessels. In addition, pastes are also a good alternative.

Acupuncture and moxibustion are also capable of up-bearing toxins. If suppuration occurs due to mistreatment or untimely treatment, toxins may have a chance to enter the interior and attack the viscera and bowels. As a result, the condition will become critical, very likely threatening life. At this juncture, the physician should support the righteous qi and bear the toxins upward to prevent them from sinking inward and further force them out. To up-bear toxins, one may perform needling to harmonize the constructive and defensive and bleeding with a three-edged needle to clear heat and dispel stasis. At the same time, it is necessary to administer some medicinals to protect the righteous qi and expel toxins. To do this, Radix Astragali Memebranacei (*Huang Qi*) is an indispensable ingredient which should be prescribed in large amounts. After such treatment, toxins will be driven from deep to superficial, and it will be easy for the sore to develop pus. When pus becomes mature, one can perform red-hot needling to open the sore and drain out this pus. Other methods, for example, cutting, may also achieve this end.

Supplementation should be used in cases of vacuity, and it becomes necessary when sores have advanced to the stage of festering. On the one hand, pus is running out, consuming the essence and blood and whittling away the righteous qi. On the other hand, the sore is eroding the flesh, while the generation of new flesh demands abundant supplies of essence and blood. At the same time, the patient may be listless and languishing. In view of all this, to heal the sore, the physician has no other way but to supplement. To supplement, one has to focus on the spleen and stomach. The stomach is the sea of water and grain, and the spleen is the source of generation and transformation. Only when these are replenished can qi and blood become abundant. There is a saying that, "Life is guaranteed when stomach qi is present, but death is a certainty when it is absent."

Supplementation takes time and its effects are slow to show themselves. To supplement, in many cases, we prefer moxibustion to needling, although needling cannot be given up altogether as a bad choice in all cases. Many acupuncturists prefer a combined therapy of needling and moxibustion to draw on the curative advantages of both. Among the indispensable points, *Zu San Li* (St 36) should be given priority. It very strongly supplements the spleen and stomach.

In sum, for external troubles, there are three remedial methods appropriate to their early, advanced, and late stages respectively: 1) dispersion of toxins in the early stage, 2) upbearing of toxins in the advanced stage, and 3) supplementation in the late stage.

In terms of different patterns, for a yin pattern, moxibustion is a better choice in most cases, while for a yang pattern, either needling or moxibustion is a good option. A vacuity pattern requires supplementation, and for supplementing one can use either moxibustion or needling. To treat a cold pattern, moxibustion is prefered. To cure a heat repletion pattern, needling is used. For a blood repletion pattern, bleeding with a three-edged needle is particularly good.

5
Needling Methods

Although there are a variety of supplementing hand techniques or manipulations in relation to acupuncture, acupuncture is particularly good at draining. Therefore, it is effective in quickening the blood and transforming stasis, clearing heat and resolving toxins, dispersing swelling and scattering nodulation, stopping pain and checking itching. In a sense, it is quicker than medication in coursing the channels and network vessels and for supporting the righteous and dispelling evils. Therefore, it is a proven fact that even for some internal disorders with heat repletion patterns, for example, appendicitis, needling may be a satisfactory alternative making expensive and complicated surgery unnecessary.

Obtaining the qi

Fine or filiform needles are the most commonly used of the nine needles. In manipulating this type of needle, one should try to obtain the qi. This is a special needling sensation which is a result of the needle stimulating the channel qi. If one locates the point accurately, qi may be obtained immediately after one inserts the needle to the right depth in the right direction. When qi comes, the practitioner will feel the needle in the patient's flesh become heavy, tight, or resistant to turning, while the patient will feel pressure, numbness, distention, or an electric sensation around the tip of the needle. This sensation may radiate or extend away to a certain distant part along the respective channel.

Traditionally, Chinese needling lays great store on obtaining the qi. *The Spiritual Pivot* says, "The key in needling is to induce qi to come, and, unless it comes, there will be no effect." The *Zhen Jiu Da Cheng (The Great Compendium of Acupuncture & Moxibustion, Great Compendium* hereinafter) by Yang Ji-zhou published in 1601 CE says, "The more swiftly the qi comes, the more swiftly the effect is brought," and, "If qi fails to come in the end, the case is beyond cure." Modern Chinese practice proves that there are cases which show effect even if the qi is not obtained. However, the fact should not be denied that there is a certain relation between the curative effect and the obtainment of the qi.

Reasons for failing to obtain the qi:

Qi failing to come may be explained by the following factors:

1. Inaccurate location of the point
2. Needle insertion to an inappropriate depth or in the wrong direction
3. Inadequate needling manipulation and/or inadequate length of stimulation
4. Vacuity of qi and blood of the patient
5. The special physique of the patient

Techniques for hastening the qi:

If the needling sensation or qi does not come when it should, one may apply one or two of the following manipulation techniques. These are called "hastening the qi (*cui qi*)."

1. Twirling: Turn the needle to the left and right.

2. Lifting & thrusting: Repeatedly withdraw the needle backward a little and then push it inward to the original depth in a small amplitude.

3. Stroking: Gently rub the skin with the fingers along the route of the needled channel.

4. Scraping: Make the needle vibrate in a small amplitude by scraping its handle with the nail of the forefinger or the thumb.

5. Rocking: Hold the upper end of the needle with the fingers and rock it about.

6. Flicking: Gently strike the body of the needle repeatedly with the fingernail.

The first two are the main techniques for hastening the qi or inducing the qi, while the others serve as aids when qi refuses to come after a comparatively long time of inducing the qi.

Draining & supplementing techniques

Draining technique and supplementing technique are special maneuvers whose purpose is to drain repletion and supplement vacuity respectively. However, before applying draining or supplementing, one should have an idea about the functions of the acupoints. Many points, like *Tian Shu* (St 25) and *Nei Guan* (Per 6), have a dual function, *i.e.*, they can be needled to drain or supplement depending upon the technique applied. Points like *Zu San Li* (St 36), *Guan Yuan* (CV 4), *Qi Hai* (CV 6), and *Bai Hui* (GV 20) are mainly supplementing in nature. That is to say that, unless one performs a special draining technique, they always play the role of supplementation. The last group, including, for instance, the Twelve Well points, the Ten Diffusing points (*Shi Xuan*, M-UE-1-5), the *Ba Xie*, (M-UE-22) in the webs between the fingers, and *Wei Zhong* (Bl 40), are distinguished for their particular effect of draining evil wind, fire heat, and toxins.

The conventional draining and supplementing hand techniques are as follows:

1. Twirling method: After obtaining the qi, if one turns the needle slowly and gently within the range of 180°, this is supplementing. On the contrary, if one turns the needle with a big force and rapidly in a range exceeding 180°, this is draining.

2. Lifting & thrusting method: After obtaining the qi, if one thrusts the needle deeper with more force and then raises it with less force, moving it deeper and deeper, this is supplementing. If one thrusts the needle with less force but lifts it with more force, moving it more and more shallowly, this is draining.

3. Varying the speed method: Slow insertion and quick extraction of the needle is supplementing, while quick insertion and slow extraction is draining.

4. Respiration method: Insertion of the needle while the patient is exhaling and extraction of it while the patient is inhaling is supplementing. Insertion of the needle while the patient is inhaling and extraction of it while the patient is exhaling is draining.

5. Opening & shutting method: Slow withdrawal of the needle and rubbing the point hole immediately upon extraction is supplementing, while quickly withdrawing the needle and leaving the needle hole open or widening the needle hole by rocking the needle in the course of extracting it is draining.

6. Direction method: Inserting the needle in the direction of the needled channel flow is supplementing, while inserting it in the direction opposite to the channel flow is draining.

Fire-needling

A thick filiform or three-edged needle is often used in fire-needling or red-hot needling (*huo zhen*) for the treatment of sores and certain other diseases. In Chinese medicine, a red-hot needle is a tool as good as the scalpel in modern surgery. It is used in opening swellings to drain pus or to directly drain toxins in curing diseases like hemorrhoids, acne, scrofula, and gangrene. Sometimes, a Chinese practitioner may prefer a red-hot knife, for example, in stripping warts for the sake of easy and convenient manipulation.

The requirements for fire-needling are steadiness, accuracy, and speed. After heating the needle to red-hot, the practitioner should swiftly insert it into the desired place and then extract it with the same rapid speed. During the operation, the hand must hold the needle steadily the whole while. An inexperienced practitioner, who is liable to get nervous at the sight of a red-hot needle, blunders involuntarily, the hand trembling and unable to hit the right place. Practically speaking, if done properly, this is quite a safe method. It damages no healthy tissue and leaves no scar or infection.

The three-edged needle

The three-edged needle with which to let out blood by pricking the blood vein is another type of needle which is often used in the treatment of external troubles. It is particularly recommended for its quick or instantaneous effects of clearing heat and resolving toxins, quickening the blood and transforming stasis, freeing the flow of the network vessels and dispersing swelling. This type of needle is used in the following five ways:

1. Needling the network vessels: The so-called network vessels are in actuality fine, protruding blood veins. The sites punctured may or may not be acupoints. This method of puncturing is good for phlebitis and varicosities for example.

2. Tip needling: This needling method is applied to the tips of the fingers and toes, *i.e.*, the twelve well points and the ten diffusing points (*Shi Xuan*, M-UE-1-5).

3. Dispersed needling: This method is often applied in comparatively extensive lesions, for instance, dropsy, hematoma, and ecchymosis. This method is so named because the points punctured are dotted all over the affected area. This method is also indicated for some other troubles, like acne. To treat acne, it is necessary to puncture several points on the upper back.

4. Cluster needling: This is also called dense needling and is applicable in problems like herpes zoster and obstinate ringworm. The treatment of such diseases requires selection of a group of points close to each other.

5. Fiber-severing: This is also known as root-cutting. It is often employed in treating acne, hemorrhoids, hives, lymphadenopathy, etc. Traditionally, the severing method consists of pricking at and breaking off the subcutaneous fibers at certain acupoints on the back or at small reactive spots on the skin which have become abnormally discolored gray, pale, red, or brown.

The cutaneous needle

The cutaneous needle, also called the plum blossom or seven star needle, is good at harmonizing the qi and blood and disinhibiting the channels and quickening the network vessels. It is effective for extensive skin problems, such as itching and numbness. Cutaneous needling can also be confined to one or more points, as in the case of headache, requiring the needling *Tou Wei* (St 8), or insect bite, which warrants needling the *a shi* point, *e.g.*, the bitten place. Or it may be performed along a related channel or a particular line, as in the case of paraplegia where the governing vessel and the paravertebral lines are needled. It may also be applied in an area, as in the case of neurodermatitis and sprain.

In manipulating the cutaneous needle, a good practitioner mainly uses their wrist to tap the skin with an even force at an even speed, making sure that the needles fall vertically. Depending on the goal of treatment, cutaneous needling may end with three different immediate consequences: reddening of the skin, blood seeping, or slight bleeding.

Auricular acupuncture

Auricular acupuncture has undergone an unsual course of evolution. Mention of needling the ears was indeed found in a number of old Chinese medical classics, but it was not until modern times that it has come into wide use. Its scope of clinical application encompasses many categories of internal disease, such as mental disorders, as well as external diseases, including dermatoses such as hives, acne, vitiligo, eczema, and psoriasis. In addition, nearly all pain conditions fall within the scope of its indications: gall and kidney stones, intestinal gripping pain, bone fracture, and soft tissue lesions. In the past, there were two troubles in applying ear acupuncture. One was difficulty in locating the right point accurately, and the other was the pain it provoked. The recently invented ear needle with its various accesories has been universally acknowledged as "a miracle-working needle." These new needles have facilitated manipulation and promoted ear acupuncture's application in a still wider field because they have solved the above two problems. Interestingly, the author has discovered that many patients who are afraid of trying ordinary acupuncture are willing to accept ear acupuncture, since they say it seems much safer.

In relation to ear acupuncture, Chinese point selection adopted nowadays is based on the following four principles:

1. Choose the corresponding points: For example, Ankle (MA-AH-2) for ankle sprain and Heart (MA) for cardiac disease.

2. Choose points according to pattern discrimination: For instance, Lung (MA-IC-1) for dermatosis because the skin is governed by the lungs. Or we may select Heart (MA) for insomnia because the heart governs the spirit. Yet again, we may choose Kidneys (MA) to treat baldness since the hair on the head is ascribed to the kidneys.

3. Choose empirical points: For example, bleeding the tip of the earlobe to abate fever.

4. Choose points based on modern Western medicine: For example, Endocrine (MA) to treat acne and Sympathetic (MA-AH-7) for disorders of some internal organs.

Electroacupuncture

Electroacupuncture is prefered by most Chinese acupuncturists today. This kind of acupuncture not only saves labor and easily controls the force of stimulation, but it also makes use of the special effects of electricity on the human body. In China, electroacupuncture is applied in nearly all cases indicating acupuncture. The cathode pole is usually attached to the main or ruling point, while the anode pole is attached to the auxiliary point. The average length of needle retention is

10 minutes. The volume of electricity should be increased gradually to the maximum. In ordinary cases, this ranges around 2 amperes, 2-5 volts, while for anesthesia it may be as large as 25 amperes, 40 volts. The frequency is usually 50-100 Hz but can be reduced to 2-5 Hz. High frequency is used to relieve pain, tranquilize the nerves, and relax muscular tension and hypertonicity of the blood vessels. Low frequency, which produces strong stimulation, gives a satisfactory effect on such problems as atony and atrophy. Alternating low and high frequency is good for improving metabolism and blood circulation and hence is geared to relieving pain and treating such troubles as sprains and frostbite. Intermittent waves are often also applied. These are able to enhance the excitability of tissues in the treatment of paraplegia, wilting, etc.

Water needle

Water needle or point injection is the product of combining the old needling art with modern Western medicine's block therapy. Since Chinese acupuncturists are free from legal restriction in using any modern medical means, they sometimes use point injection therapy. The routine procedures and requirements are similar to those of block therapy. The points should be few in number, and the injected solution may be made from Chinese medicinals or modern Western medicine. Although such water needling can be very effective, such point injection with "hollow" needles is typically outside the legal scope of practice of non-MD acupuncturists in most Western countries.

6
Methods of Moxibustion

The Spiritual Pivot says, "When the blood is congealed, settling in the vessels, there is no way to remove it except through rectifying (the blood) by fire." In another place, it says:

> If the vessel is sunken, there is blood binding within. When there is retarded blood and blood cold, it is appropriate to apply moxibustion.

These instructions imply that moxibustion is the best choice specifically for warming the channels, scattering cold, and harmonizing the qi and blood.

Clinically, moxibustion has a very broad scope of application, including internal problems, external troubles, gynecology, pediatrics, dermatology, etc. It is often resorted to in treating chronic diseases, but many emergency cases also fall within its indications, for instance, syncope and shock. Not only is it able to heal mild maladies, but it cures recalcitrant, enduring diseases such as lymphadenitis and bedsores. Moxibustion also often has a miraculous effect on various external sores and superficial traumas. Once the author met with a case of double tongue, a swelling on the underside of the tongue. Using a moxa roll, I moxaed over *Lian Quan* (CV 23) for some time. Unexpectedly, the swelling disappeared instantly. It is also interesting that moxibustion has long been found to be an effective aid for keeping fit and preventing disease. *The Thousand (Pieces of) Gold* says:

> People who tour Wu and Shu should moxa some points (regularly) and leave the sores unhealed for some time. This will keep the toxic qi of miasma, leprosy, and warm malaria away from them.

Wu refers to the coastal areas of southeast China, while Shu is now Sichuan province. In olden times, these were frontier areas. *The Great Compendium* also says, "If one intends to be safe and sound, one should keep *San Li* (St 36) wet (from the drainage of a moxibustion sore)." Nowadays it is well-known that moxibustion is a good means to treat and prevent such diseases as hypertension and colds.

The flavors, nature & functions of Artemisia Argyium

As regards the issue of why, of all medicinals, Folium Artemisiae Argyii (*Ai Ye*) has always been chosen for moxibustion above any others, many past outstanding medical men have given their explanations. In his *Ben Cao Cong Xin (Newly Collated Materia Medica)*, Wu Yi-luo, who lived in the Qin dynasty, the last imperial dynasty in China, gives a typical account, saying:

> Mugwort is bitter and acrid in flavor and is able to generate heat. It is pure yang in nature. Therefore, it is able to recover expired yang. It reaches all the twelve channels, penetrates the three yin (channels), rectifies the qi and blood, expels cold and dampness, and warms the uterus... When burnt, it penetrates the various channels to eliminate the hundreds of diseases.

Below is a description of the various methods of moxibustion.

Methods of moxibustion:

Moxa cones

Cone moxibustion was the commonly used method of moxibustion in olden times. Nowadays, its use is limited. However, some practitioners still do prefer it. Such cones can be as large as a plum or as small as a grain of wheat depending upon the degree of severity and extent of the disease. Before it is made into cones, the mugwort, which must be of high quality, should have been seasoned for more than nine years. This storing and drying results in the evaporation of much of its oils, and, therefore, it burns moderately and will not damage the skin. Mugwort cones can be set directly over a point, *i.e.*, in touch with the skin, or over salt, garlic, ginger, etc. Depending on its immediate result, moxibustion is classified into the following types:

1. Scarring moxibustion

Scarring moxibustion refers to the burning of the required number of cones, one by one, directly on the skin and then leaving the burn(s) untreated. A couple of days later, the blister(s) will burst and then heal, leaving a scar. This technique is suitable for intractable tubercular lymphadenopathy, enduring ulceration, etc. The blister and its sore thus caused are called a moxibustion flower. In former times and still by some practitioners, the production of such a moxa flower has been considered crucial for successful treatment. The *Tai Ping Sheng Hui Fang (The Sagelike Formulas from the Tai Ping [Era], Sagelike Formulas* hereinafter) published in 992 CE says:

> Suppose a sufficient number of cones are burned up. Only when a sore develops and weeps pus may the disease be cured. If no sore is produced or no pus engendered, the disease will not be relieved.

In modern times, some Chinese practitioners continue with this practice, and their clinical experience confirms that intentionally produced moxa sores do have something to do with the curative effect.

In spite of its effectiveness, only a few patients are undaunted enough to receive this therapy because of the pain it inflicts. To reduce the pain, the *Bian Que Xin Shu (Bian Que's Heart Book)* published in 1146 CE suggested prescribing a sleeping formula before the treatment, while the author of the *Shou Shi Bao Yuan (Prolong Life by Protecting the Origin)*, Gong Ting-xian (1522-1619 CE), invented a finger pressing method to induce local anesthesia. For local anesthesia, modern Chinese practitioners have anesthetics at their service, while others simply use their palms to clap the skin to be moxaed to induce anesthesia.

2. Non-scarring moxibustion

Non-scarring moxibustion refers to the technique whereby the burning cone is changed with a new one as soon as it has burnt to the extent that it causes a burning heat to the skin. This moxibustion method does not produce blisters but barely reddens the skin. It is often employed in such cases as ringworm, eczema, and enduring internal diseases.

Lying between the above two methods, there is another method called blister moxibustion. This moxibustion method may cause a slight burn which develops into a blister a short time later but does not go on to develop a weeping sore. This method can be used for acne, scrofula, and vitiligo.

3. Indirect moxibustion

The method of cone moxibustion used most commonly in China today involves moxaing over a layer or a thin slice of garlic, salt, medicated cake, ginger, or scallion. The substance, such as garlic, can be mashed for this purpose. In terms of the extent to which such moxibustion should be performed, there is a short passage in *The Orthodox Gathering* which says:

> To treat any species of sore at its onset...set a thin slice of garlic over the sore, burning three cones over (the garlic one after the other)... If pain is felt before moxaing, moxibustion should be continued until the pain has given way to a sort of itching. If there is no pain before moxaing, the moxibustion should continue until pain and itching come... If the moxa cones (thus burned) fail to bring the desired result, it is necessary to dab (the sore) with mashed garlic, over which spread mugwort. Then burn the mugwort. At any rate, no (curative) effect will result unless (the moxibustion) causes pain. This shows that the fire qi has penetrated internally and that all the flesh is necrotic above the depth of the place where the pain is felt.

Moxa roll

Most modern Chinese practitioners prefer to use a moxa roll. This moxibustion method is painless and, therefore, all patients are willing to accept it. The roll can be held above the place to be moxaed and moved vertically up and down or in a circle. The former is called sparrow-pecking moxibustion, while the latter is called circling moxibustion. There is another method known as pressing moxibustion. In that case, the steps are to spread a piece of cloth or paper over the site of disease. Next, the burning end of a medicated or moxa roll is placed on this paper or cloth for a moment. Then the roll is swiftly removed. If the roll is made very thin, such moxibustion can be done without the paper or cloth. This is known as flash-moxibustion. This causes a beneficial, slight burning of the skin.

Heavenly moxibustion

Heavenly moxibustion, also known as paste moxibustion, is a method analogous to imbedding a needle in acupuncture. Though so named, it neither involves mugwort nor burning. In practice, it refers to the application of a paste made from an herbal medicinal or a mixture of medicinals. The medicinals commonly used for such pastes include Semen Sinapis Albae (*Bai Jie Zi*), Mylabris (*Ban Mao*), Bulbus Allii Sativi (*Da Suan*), Radix Euphobiae Kansui (*Gan Sui*), Semen Strychnotis (*Ma Qian Zi*), Herba Menthae Haplocalycis (*Bo He*), Semen Ricini Communis (*Bi Ma Zi*), Radix Clematidis Chinensis (*Wei Ling Xian*), Fructus Evodiae Rutecarpae (*Wu Zhu Yu*), Herba Asari Cum Radice (*Xi Xin*), and uncooked Radix Lateralis Aconiti Carmichaeli (*Sheng Fu Zi*). The majority of such medicinals are irritating and may provoke pain or even blistering on contact with the skin.

7
Cupping

In olden times, cupping was named horning. This old name apparently suggests that this method was invented very long ago, before such utensils as cups were made. At first, it was mainly used to help remove pus when treating sores and swellings. Later, its clinical application gradually expanded to include a number of other external troubles as well as certain internal disorders. Cupping has the peculiar advantage of directly drawing out evils, such as cold and dampness, through the channels as well as toxins from, for instance, snake bite, cinnabar fire, and clove sores. Therefore, nowadays, it is widely used in many kinds of external troubles. Moreover, since something can be found as a cupping tool in any house, for example, a cup or a piece of bamboo, and its operation is simple and convenient, many laypersons perform cupping in their homes for illnesses which are not thought serious. Cupping as an aid to self-cure is especially popular in the countryside where many people cannot afford to pay for health care and where, equally importantly, there is a lack of qualified physicians.

In doing cupping, one can use one or a number of cups. In other words, one can perform cupping over one or a number of points depending on the number and extent of the lesions. After applying the cup, the cup is usually retained in position for some time. Below is a description of several other cupping methods:

1. Sliding cupping

This method is used on places where the flesh is thick and the trouble is extensive, for example, migratory wind damp pain. Before doing the cupping, one should apply oil over the surface of the skin. Then, after the cup is made fixed over the point, gently push it to and fro some distance without allowing any air to get into the cup, thus breaking the vacuum seal. Usually this is done over the affected area itself or along a section of the route of the affected channel.

2. Flash-cupping

Fix the cup over the intended site and then remove it immediately. Do this repeatedly over the same place until reddening of the skin appears.

3. Combined needling & cupping

A point is punctured and then one does cupping over that point after the needle has been withdrawn or sometimes while the needle is still in position. This is particularly effective for wind damp impediment (previously simply called *bi*) pain. A variant of this method is cupping after bleeding by pricking with a bleeding or three-edged needle. This is intended to produce even more bleeding.

4. Medicinal cupping

The simple method of medicinal cupping is to dip or boil cups made from sections of bamboo in a medicinal solution before they are used for cupping. Another way is to insert a bag containing certain medicinals inside the cup before applying it. This bag is then retained inside the cup and comes in contact with the skin once it is in place. This method is often used in such internal disorders as asthma, cough, colds, ulceration, gastritis, and indigestion as well as for some external troubles like wind damp impediment pain and psoriasis.

8
A Guide to Point Selection

The difference between the acupuncture-moxibustion treatment of external troubles and that of internal disorders is that local points should be given more consideration in the former. Apart from that, the principles of point selection are the same, *i.e.*, points should be chosen in accordance with the involved channel(s) and network vessel(s), the condition of the viscera and bowels, and the vacuity and repletion of the qi and blood.

Acupuncture and moxibustion are a medical modality for bringing effect through the stimulation of points. This peculiarity of acupuncture and moxibustion makes proper point selection of paramount importance. There are three ways of selecting points and these have undergone no change over the thousands of years of the existence of this therapy.

1. Local selection

The selection of local points involves the stimulation of local *a shi* points. These are tender places or places of pressure pain right in the immediate area of the trauma, sore, swelling, etc. Such local points are often the focus in handling external troubles. For a number of external troubles, choosing only local points is sufficient. Moxaing *a shi* points alone to treat tennis elbow is a good example, while hemorrhoids may merely require applying red-hot needling as another extreme example.

2. Proximate selection

Proximate selection means choosing points around or in the neighboring area of the lesion. The points selected may be located on a channel or may simply be *a shi* points. For instance, to treat bedsores or alopecia, one should use peripheral needling. This means needling all around the periphery of the lesion. This is one method of proximate selection.

3. Distant selection

Distant selection refers to choosing from the five transport points and other such major points below the elbows and knees. Distant points are usually selected based on the generalized signs and symptoms. Selection of such distant points aims at freeing the channels, harmonizing the viscera and bowels, and balancing the constructive and defensive. Distant selection should also include points specific for certain generalized signs or symptoms, since even the same named diseases may differ from one another in their manifestations. Therefore, even if we are faced with the same external disease, we may have to vary our prescription of points, which may be few or many in number. For example, in a case of carbuncles, if there is the complication of fever, we should choose *Da Zhui* (GV 14). If, on the other hand, there is retching and vomiting, *Nei Guan* (Per 6) should be needled.

Since even diseases which seem simple at first glance may involve more than one part of the body and display more than one sign or symptom, the above three ways of point selection are often combined to treat a single problem.

Ruling & auxiliary points

Point selection is a matter that demands prudence, knowledge, and experience. Although the distinction of sovereign, minister, assistant, and envoy used in the design of medicinal formulas is not used in point selection, an effective point combination consists of one or two ruling or main points plus some secondary or auxiliary points which work well synergistically with the ruling ones. While the choice of ruling point is extremely important, even the selection of a different auxiliary point may bring about a radically different result. Suppose *He Gu* (LI 4), an important point for rectifying the qi, is chosen as the ruling point. It is able to upbear and downbear, to open and diffuse. Supoose *Qu Chi* (LI 11) is chosen as its assistant. It is able to clear heat and dispel wind, harmonize the constructive and defensive, and quicken the blood and resolve the muscles. This is a wonderful combination to rectify the upper burner and heal various types of dermatoses. If, instead, *San Yin Jiao* (Sp 6) is chosen as the auxiliary point, because it is able to rectify the qi and regulate the menses, then this combination is a good formula for gynecological problems. If the auxiliary point is *Fu Liu* (Ki 7), then these points will resolve and consolidate the exterior as well as harmonize the constructive and defensive. If *Tai Chong* (Liv 3) is combined with *He Gu* (LI 4), then these two have the ability to track down wind and unblock impediment, move stasis and free the channels, open the portals and arouse the spirit. This latter combination of ruling and auxiliary points is called the four gates or bars. In this context, the word gate (*guan*) implies a wide coverage of indications and frequent use.

Other methods of point combination

The methods of point combination in common use are as follows:

1. Combination of local & distant points

This method of point combining gives equal importance to attacking the localized lesion and improving the state of the body as a whole. The local point(s) is or are to remove toxins directly from the lesion, while the distant point(s), which is/are located on the relevant channel(s), serve to free flow of the channel as well as the qi and blood. For example, *San Li* (St 36) may be chosen to treat welling abscess on the front of the neck, but *Kun Lun* (Bl 60) should be chosen to treat welling abscess on the back of the neck.

2. Combination of points above & below

Above and below can mean several different things. They may refer to points above and below the lesion, points on the upper and lower limbs, and points at the two ends of a relevant channel. For example, to treat stiffness of the head and the back of the neck, we may choose *Lie Que* (Lu 7) on the forearm in combination with *Fu Yang* (Bl 59) which is located on the foot. To heal hemorrhoids, one may needle *Yin Jiao* (CV 7) and *Chang Qiang* (GV 1) which are located far apart. To restore prolapsed rectum, *Chang Qiang* (GV 1) and *Bai Hui* (GV 20) are an ideal combination. In the case of a sprained ankle, one may perform needling at the wrist in addition to the ankle.

3. Combination of left & right

Needling points bilaterally is one example of combining points on the left and right. However, if the trouble is located unilaterally, for instance, a deviated mouth and eye, one often may have to needle pertinent points on the side opposite to the site of the disease. In yet other cases, one should treat the pertinent points on the same side as the site of the disease. This is also regarded as combining points on the left and the right.

4. Combination of front & back

According to this method of point combination for a disease on the front, one chooses points on the back in addition to those on the front or vice versa. Thus for heart pain, one may choose *Xin Shu* (Bl 15) on the back, while in the case of breast welling abscess *Ge Shu* (Bl 17) and one or more points in the neighborhood of the welling abscess. One typical combination of the front and the back is to choose an alarm point on the front and a transporting point on the back. To treat lung disorders, for example, one may needle *Zhong Fu* (Lu 1) and *Fei Shu* (Bl 13). The front alarm point and the back transporting point both have direct access to the viscus. When needled together, they have a coordinated effect of hitting the disease from opposite directions.

5. Combination of exterior & interior

Here, exterior refers to the yang channel, while interior means the yin channel. Thus, typically, in this method, points on the yang channel are combined with points on the yin channel. This method is widely used to simultaneously level or normalize the viscera and the bowels. To treat diseases of the skin, which is ascribed to the lungs, choosing *He Gu* (LI 4) and *Qu Chi* (LI 11) is also considered a combination of the exterior with the interior. *He Gu* and *Qu Chi* are both points on the large intestine channel, but the large intestine and the lungs stand in an exterior-interior relationship. Therefore, through needling *He Gu* and *Qu Chi*, the lungs are leveled or made normal and consequently the skin disease is healed.

6. Combination of channels of the same name

As an example of this method of point combining, there is a *yang ming* channel on both the upper and the lower limbs. Two such channels with the same yin-yang name are closely connected and therefore may act synergistically. To treat toothache, for instance, one may choose *He Gu* (LI 4) and *Nei Ting* (St 44). The first of these points is on the hand *yang ming* and the second is on the foot *yang ming*.

Book Two: Dermatoses & Infectious Sores

1
Introduction

Pattern discrimination

Treatment based on pattern discrimination is peculiar to Chinese medicine and acupuncture. It is based on the combined consideration of all the essential pathogenic factors and provides the basis for eradicating even recalcitrant diseases by pulling them up by the root. In clinical practice, it is not uncommon to see patients who are overjoyed to find themselves freed from some old, intractable affliction, such as stomachache, at the same time that their main complaint, for instance, some dermatosis is cured. This unexpected side effect may well be credited, at least in part, to treatment based on pattern discrimination. This is because the pattern is made up of the entirety of the patient's signs and symptoms, not just the pathognomonic systems of their main complaint or disease.

1. Disease cause pattern discrimination

In terms of Chinese medicine, like any other diseases, dermatoses and infectious cutaneous and subcutaneous sores are caused by the six environmental execesses externally, the seven affects internally and other neither internal or external causes, such as an unhealthy diet. In many cases, they are due to a conspiracy between two or more of these.

In terms of external causes, the disease causes of hives and senile pruritus are easily tracked down to wind. It is evident even to a layperson that skin cracking may be caused by dryness and heat. In sores which are accompanied by fever, thirst, spontaneous sweating, reddish, *i.e.*, dark-colored urine, and constipation, fire is found as the evil responsible. In treating such sores or rashes, the practitioner should direct their attention to the root cause—wind, fire, or dryness. It is no wonder then that when one drives the evils out, healing of the sore or rash is realized along with the elimination of any complications linked with the root cause.

In terms of internal causes, Chinese medicine lays great store in emotional factors. As an outstanding example, balding is often a product of lasting stress or depression. Neurodermatitis is another example of an emotional disorder leading to disease.

Overeating fatty, acrid, peppery, and sweet foods must also be added to the list of the disease causes in external dermatological conditions because these substances may generate heat and phlegm, and, needless to say, heat may produce toxins, in which case, sores will be caused. From the Chinese medical point of view, sores can be the result of pouring phlegm. Where phlegm settles, there is binding or nodulation, and bound phlegm will inevitably wreak havoc.

2. Channel & network vessel pattern discrimination

Pattern discrimination is the key to successful treatment, but what is its framework? Firstly, one should discriminate the pattern according to the channels. For an acupuncturist, this is not difficult to do, for such pattern discrimination is based on the routes of the channels. Sores on the back of the neck are ascribed to the governing vessel and the foot *tai yang* channel, while those on the lateral aspect of the neck are attributed to the foot *shao yang* and hand *tai yang* channels. For troubles involving the mouth and lips, the hand and foot *yang ming* and the foot *jue yin* channels are responsible.

3. Qi & blood pattern discrimination

It is not so easy to identify a pattern in relation to the qi and blood. As far as the qi is concerned, there are usually two patterns, qi vacuity and qi stagnation. Clues to the diagnosis of the qi vacuity pattern include such generalized signs and symptoms as fatigue, a low, *i.e.*, weak, voice, diminished qi, spontaneous sweating, and a fine, weak pulse. Chronic hives may present all or some of the above manifestations. The qi stagnation pattern is characterized by an intermittent sensation of distention of the affected part where nodules or a raised mass of papules are often found.

In connection with the blood, there are three basic patterns: blood vacuity, blood stasis, and blood heat. The blood vacuity pattern is verified if there is a white or sallow yellow facial complexion, dizziness, flowery, *i.e.*, blurred, vision, heart palpitations, insomnia, profuse dreaming, numbness of the extremities, coarse, thickened skin, dryness and scaling or cracking of the skin, desiccated nails, withered hair, a pale tongue, and a fine pulse. Some cases of chronic psoriasis and balding may be grouped under this pattern.

The blood stasis pattern, which is often seen in such cases as allergic purpura, hematoma, and red nodulations, is revealed by fixed pain, a dark color of the overlying skin, subcutaneous nodules, ecchymosis, and a dark-colored or purplish tongue.

The blood heat pattern is manifest by complications of bleeding, including hematuria, hemafecia, and nasal bleeding, excessive menstruation, vexation, thirst, a red tongue, a bright red color of the overlying skin, and a rapid pulse. This pattern may appear in allergic purpura, dermatitis medicamentosa, and eczema.

4. Viscera & bowel pattern discrimination

Another focus of pattern discrimination is establishing the relationships between the internal five viscera and six bowels and diseases in the exterior. First of all, in the treatment of dermatoses and sores, one should make a study of the lungs and the large intestines, since they govern the skin and hair. Concerning them there are four patterns:

A. Lung qi vacuity pattern: If chronic hives, chronic eczema, pruritus, lupus erythmatosus, scleroderma, and dermatomyositis are complicated by shortness of breath, a weak voice, fatigue, coughing with thin phlegm, spontaneous sweating, aversion to cold, a pale tongue, a white facial complexion, and a weak, floating pulse, they are classified as this pattern.

B. Lung yin vacuity pattern: This pattern is characterized by the complications of tidal fever, coughing with scanty phlegm, night sweats, withered, brittle hair, red cheeks, a red tongue body with little fur, and a rapid, fine pulse.

C. Lung channel heat pattern: Diseases like acne, drinker's nose, and seborrheic dermatitis are diagnosed as this pattern if the skin reddens along the route of the lung channel.

D. Large intestine damp heat pattern: In this pattern, there are generalized signs and symptoms of fever, thirst, abdominal pain, blood in the stools or constipation, yellow, slimy tongue fur, and a rapid, slippery pulse. Large intestine damp heat may be seen in diseases such as acute hives, herpes zoster, and allergic purpura.

In respect to the heart and small intestine, there are also four patterns pertaining dermatoses and sores:

A. Heart yin vacuity pattern: This pattern may be seen in chronic hives, ephidrosis, ulceration of the oral cavity, chronic eczema, etc. It is usually accompanied by heart palpitations, vexation, insomnia, profuse dreaming, dizziness, impaired memory, night sweats, a dry mouth, red cheeks, a red tongue with little fur, and a rapid, fine pulse.

B. Heart yang vacuity pattern: Scleroderma, measles, Raynaud's disease, etc. may all present this pattern if they are accompanied by heart palpitations, spirit abstraction, shortness of breath, generalized weakness, pain and oppression in the chest, cold limbs, swollen limbs and face, a purplish green-blue color of the fingers and toes, a white facial complexion, a pale tongue with white fur, and a deep, slow pulse.

C. Heart blood stasis pattern: Besides many of the same generalized signs and symptoms as in the pattern immediately above, this pattern is distinguished by the intermittency of its symptoms, a dark, purple tongue with static spots, green-blue lips, and a deep, choppy pulse.

D. Small intestine damp heat pattern: The characteristic features of this pattern that aid in its diagnosis are short voidings of scanty urine, thirst and a desire for water, mouth ulcers, a red face, a red tongue, and a rapid pulse.

The disease causes of qi stagnation and depression are associated with the liver and gallbladder. Five patterns of dermatoses and sores are connected with this viscus and bowel:

A. Liver qi depression & binding pattern: A dermatosis or sore may be safely diagnosed as this pattern if it is accompanied by such generalized signs and symptoms as rib-side (previously translated as lateral costal) distention and fullness, lower abdominal pain and distention, vexation, agitation, irascibility, dizziness, menstrual irregularity, painful menstruation, insomnia, profuse dreaming, thin tongue fur, and a bowstring pulse.

B. Effulgent liver fire pattern: This pattern is characterized by such generalized signs and symptoms as vexation, irascibility, a red face, red, swollen eyes, a bitter taste in the mouth, thirst, constipation, yellow or reddish urine, a red tongue body with yellow fur, and a rapid, bowstring pulse.[1]

C. Liver channel cold dampness pattern: Because dampness is inclined to pour downward and because the liver channel wraps the genitals, this pattern is characterized by contraction of the scrotum, lower abdominal pain, and ulcerated genitals with itching.

D. Liver blood vacuity pattern: The generalized signs and symptoms which aid in the diagnosis of this pattern include dizziness, dryness of the eyes, flowery, *i.e.*, blurred, vision, dry, brittle hair, numbness of the limbs, dryness of the skin, a dry, cracked tongue, and a weak, fine pulse.

E. Liver-gallbladder damp heat pattern: Dermatoses and sores characterized as this pattern are accompanied by jaundice, rib-side distention and pain, a bitter taste in the mouth, thirst, red eyes,

---

[1] Wiseman gives stringlike pulse for *xian mai*. However, the character contains the bow radical and the pulse image has a taut quality like a bowstring. In other words, it is not like a loose or limp string. Wiseman's previous translation for this pulse quality was wiry. He changed this to stringlike since Chinese were not technologically able to manufacture wire at the time this term was originally coined.

abdominal distention, torpid intake, reddish urine, slimy yellow tongue fur, and a slippery, bowstring pulse.

However, the majority of diseases are closely related with the spleen and stomach because they are the source of generation and transformation or the root of latter heaven or postnatal qi. When this viscus and bowel are involved in dermatoses and sores, they may exhibit the following patterns:

A. Spleen qi vacuity pattern: This pattern may manifest swelling and edema, a sallow yellow facial complexion, fatigue, and low food intake.

B. Spleen bood vacuity pattern: Bleeding, such as hematuria, ejection of blood (*i.e.*, nosebleed, hemoptysis, and hematemesis), and subcutaneous bleeding, is an important feature of this pattern. In addition, there is fatigue, listlessness, heart palpitations, shortness of breath, dizziness, a somber white or sallow yellow facial complexion, and profuse menstrual flow in women. In actuality, this pattern is spleen qi not containing the blood.

C. Spleen-stomach vacuity cold pattern: This pattern manifests as a cold body, fatigue, aversion to cold, abdominal pain relievable by pressure, abdominal distention, diarrhea, low food intake, a pale tongue with white fur, and a deep, slippery pulse.

D. Central qi fall pattern: Because the central qi has fallen below and is unable to upbear and lift in turn due to qi vacuity, there may be prolapse of the rectum or uterus or sagging of the internal organs. Dyspneic difficult breathing may arise on the slightest movement with a somber white facial complexion, aching in the limbs, disinclination to move, and swollen limbs. There may also be hematuria and hemafecia due to the spleen qi not containing the blood.

E. Stomach & intestines damp heat pattern: The generalized signs and symptoms that aid in the diagnosis of this pattern of dermatoses and sores include abdominal distention and pain exacerbated by the slightest pressure, bad breath, constipation, thirst and a desire for cold drinks, swift digestion with rapid hungering, a red tongue with slimy, yellow fur, and a rapid, slippery pulse.

The last pair of viscera and bowels are the kidneys and urinary bladder. The kidneys are the root of the heaven or prenatal qi, and in them is stored the source qi of the whole body. When the kidneys and bladder are involved, the following patterns may appear:

A. Kidney yin vacuity pattern: Kidney yin vacuity manifests as ringing in the ears, dizziness, a dry throat, profuse dreaming, insomnia, night sweats, seminal emission, aching and flaccid low back and knees, a dry tongue and mouth, a red tongue with little fur, a rapid, fine pulse, and distressed heat in the five hearts, *i.e.*, the heart, the soles of the feet, and the palms of the hands.

B. Kidney yang vacuity pattern: When there is an insufficiency of kidney yang, a cold body, aching low back, ringing in the ears, seminal emission, impotence, abdominal pain, diarrhea, swollen limbs, a pale tongue with white, thin fur, and a deep, weak pulse may appear.

C. Bladder damp heat pattern: If damp heat pours downward, urinary urgency, frequent voiding of urine, low back pain, pain in the penis (in men), fever, a dry mouth, a red tongue with thick, slimy fur, and a rapid, slippery pulse will appear.

2
Nodulations (Furuncles)

Disease causes, disease mechanisms

A furuncle, which is called a nodulation (*jie*) in Chinese medicine, is an acute, inflammatory sore. In the classics, there is no lack of descriptions of this disease. *The Origins* says:

> The swelling is 1-2 *cun* (in diameter) and is named a node. It looks like a welling abscess, a heat welling abscess. Over time, it will develop pus and open. It will heal when its pus and (decayed) blood has run out. It is also wind heat qi which settles in the skin that gives rise to the node as a result of congestion and binding of the qi and blood.

In his *Zheng Zhi Zhun Sheng (The Norms of Patterns & Their Treatment, Norms* hereinafter) released in 1602 CE, Wang Ken-tang said:

> At first the node is a protuberance, floating with no root or feet. It is a swelling of less than 2-3 *cun* in diameter within the skin. It gives a slight pain. In several days, it softens a little, and a thin layer of the (overlying) skin scales, giving off a clear fluid. Later it may become open with pus running out.

As to the disease causes, *Sagelike Formulas* says:

> Nodes are generated by blood binding and gathering which arises when wind, damp, and cold qi contend in the blood. When people are on a long travel or laboring, the yang qi diffuses and drains out due to the discharge of sweat. If they are caught in cold damp qi, this cold and dampness will contend in the channels and network vessels. After meeting with cold, blood is thwarted, becoming bound and stagnant, blocking (the channels and network vessels). Thus a node arises.

The above quotes all deal with the external causes of nodulations or rather external affection by the six environmental excesses. As regards their internal causes, this disease is usually impugned to dry heat of the viscera and bowels and disharmony of the qi and blood. In some cases, the root cause may be pure heat wasting thirst. In other cases, it is sexual taxation, emotional disturbance, or a diet of fat meat, fine grains, and rich dainties in particular. Sweet food is liable to produce fullness in the center, and fat generates heat. As a result, impairment of spleen movement and transformation arises. Then the viscera and bowels become dry and hot. Yin fire becomes fulminant, wasting and burning stomach yin. Hence the fluids and humors fail to give efflorescence (*i.e.*, provide nourishment) to the muscles and skin. As heat qi settles in the muscles and skin, the flow of the constructive and defensive becomes sluggish. Since the constructive is too vacuous to perform its function, *i.e.*, nourishing the skin, while the defensive is too vacuous to defend the exterior, evils find a chance to invade.

Types of nodulations

There are several types of nodulations in Chinese external medicine. These are named for their location, shape, some other peculiarity, or time of occurrence.

1. Summerheat nodulations

This category, also called heat nodulations or fire nodulations, occurs in summer and autumn. In most cases, they appear on the face and head, particularly in children. In hot, stuffy weather, sweat cannot exit freely. Therefore, damp heat lodges in the interstices, obstructing the flow of qi and blood and thus giving rise to miliaria. Unable to bear the itching, the small child scratches and infection ensues.

2. Mole cricket nodulations

As a matter of fact, this nodulation is shaped like the hole of the mole cricket, long and with connected protuberances. This develops from a summerheat nodulation, usually on the head of a small child. If a summerheat nodulation is not treated properly or is scratched, toxins may penetrate deeper and spread under the skin, eroding the flesh and skin and giving rise to the mole cricket nodulation.

Treatment principles: Clear heat and resolve toxins, cool the blood and disperse swelling. Choose pertinent points on the yang channels as the ruling ones.

Formula: *Ling Tai* (GV 10), *Da Zhui* (GV 14), and *Wei Zhong* (Bl 40)

Treatment method: Needle using draining technique. It is better to prick the last two points with a three-edged needle.

Explanation of the formula: *Da Zhui* (GV 14) is the meeting point of the various yang channels and is therefore, miraculous at clearing heat toxins. *Ling Tai* (GV 10) is a proven effective point for various sores. *Wei Zhong* (BL 40) is a particularly good point for clearing heat and cooling the blood.

Other choices:

1. Insert two needles crosswise transversely under the base of the furuncle. However, cross-needling is prohibited on the face.

2. Prick *Shen Zhu* (GV 12) or *Wei Zhong* (Bl 40) with a three-edged needle to let a drop of blood out.

3. Moxibustion may be applied in all stages of this disease and is especially effective for suppuration. Direct or indirect moxibustion, for example, over garlic, ginger, or with a mugwort cigar, is OK.

4. Apply pastes externally over the nodulation, such as *Ba Du Gao* (Outdraw Toxins Paste) which is commercially available in China. This formula is composed of 3.2 *liang* of the following ingredients:

Radix Ampelopsis Japonicae (*Bai Lian*)
Rhizoma Atractylodis (*Cang Zhu*)
Fructus Forsythiae Suspensae (*Lian Qiao*)
Radix Scutellariae Baicalensis (*Huang Qin*)
Radix Angelicae Dahuricae (*Bai Zhi*)
Semen Momordicae Cochinensis (*Mu Bie Zi*)
Squama Manitis Pentadactylis (*Chuan Shan Jia*)
Radix Rubrus Paeoniae Lactiflorae (*Chi Shao*)
Fructus Gardeniae Jasminoidis (*Zhi Zi*)
Radix Et Rhizoma Rhei (*Da Huang*)
Semen Ricini Communis (*Bi Ma Zi*)
Flos Lonicerae Japonicae (*Jin Yin Hua*)
uncooked Radix Rehmanniae (*Sheng Di*)
Radix Angelicae Sinensis (*Dang Gui*)
Cortex Phellodendri (*Huang Bai*)
Rhizoma Coptidis Chinensis (*Huang Lian*)

and 6 *qian* of the following ingredients:

Scolopendra Subspinipes (*Wu Gong*)
Resina Olibani (*Ru Xiang*)
Rseina Myrrhae (*Mo Yao*)
Sanguis Draconis (*Xue Jie*)
Acacia Catechu (*Er Cha*)
Calomelas (*Qing Fen*)
Camphora (*Zhang Nao*)
Hydrogyrum Oxydatum Crudum Rubrum (*Sheng Dan*)

Case history: A 24 year old male soldier had suffered from extensive mole cricket nodulations in the back of his neck and upper back for over a year. He had been treated in various ways with no effect. The lesion, quite painful, looked rugged, having several openings from which pus issued out. Combined needling and moxibustion was performed. The points needled were the same as in the formula above, while moxibustion was performed over the affected area. In each treatment, as a necessary step, *Wei Zhong* (Bl 40) was pricked to let a little blood out. One month of treatment healed the case.

References:

In a study of 45 cases of nodulation, *Feng Chi* (GB 20), *Qu Chi* (LI 11), and *Wei Zhong* (Bl 40) were needled 1 time each day using draining technique. The needles were retained for 15 minutes. Lifting and thrusting manipulation was done 3 times during needle retention to strengthen stimulation. In the course of treatment, fumigation was also employed. Of the total number of cases treated with this protocol, 41 were cured and 2 reported marked improvement. Zhou Qing-yi: *Zhong Yi Za Zhi (Journal of Chinese Medicine)* 1982; 23 (4):36.

There is also a report on the treatment of nodulations by pricking with a three-edged needle. Two points, *He Gu* (LI 4) and *Wei Zhong* (Bl 40), were both pricked bilaterally. This pricking was followed by pressing out a few drops of blood. After that, these two points were moxaed till the patient felt a little hot. An average of 2-3 treatments achieved a cure. Wang Yu-dong: *Zhe Jiang Zhong Yi Za Zhi (Zhejiang J. of C.M.)* 1990; 25 (9):423.

Supplement: Folliculitis

This is a special type of furuncle. If it occurs at the hairline on the back of the neck, it is called a hairline sore. If it occurs on the hip, it is called nightstool or bench sore. In most cases, it is due to the conspiracy of external wind and internally depressed damp heat which then transforms into fire toxins. These two evils accumulate and settle within the skin and flesh, eroding them. This disease is characterized by frequent recurrence, a long course, and multiple sites.

Treatment principles: Clear heat and resolve toxins, disperse swelling and scatter nodulation

Treatment choices:

1. Bleed *Wei Zhong* (Bl 40). The steps are to bind the knee proximal to the point (to be bled) and then prick the point with a three-edged needle to let out blood till the blood turns from dark to bright red. Treat 1 time per week.

2. Needle *Da Zhui* (GV 14), *Feng Chi* (GB 20), *Kun Lun* (Bl 60), *Da Zhong* (Ki 4), or the tender point, using draining technique.

3. Perform pricking and then cupping at *Ling Tai* (GV 10).

4. Moxa the local *a shi* point, *Da Zhui* (GV 14), *Shou San Li* (LI 10), and *Yang Lao* (SI 6).

Case history: A 25 year old male complained of folliculitis in multiple places on the back of his neck. These were so painful that they restricted the movement of his neck. The patient had been given medicine but to no effect. The prescription was to prick *Da Zhui* (GV 14) to let out about 3ml of blood. Following the bleeding, the pain and swelling disappeared. Two more treatments healed the sore.

3
Welling Abscesses

Disease causes, disease mechanisms

Welling abscesses are an important topic in nearly all the extant old classics. In his *Jing Yue Quan Shu (Jing-yue's Complete Book)* by the great scholar Zhang Jie-bin (1563-1640 CE), there is a passage describing *yong*. It says:

> Welling abscesses are the external expression of congested heat, a yang toxic qi. The swelling is serious. It is red with intense pain. The (overlying) skin is thin and lustrous. It easily develops a water blister, and, (once open,) it easily closes. It comes as swiftly as it heals.

Welling abscesses are usually accompanied by few generalized symptoms. Sometimes, the patient may suffer from fever and chills and thirst.

Types of welling abscesses

There are a variety of types of welling abscesses. These are usually named for their position, for example, umbilical welling abscesses and hip welling abscesses. The following is a brief discussion of commonly encountered types of welling abscesses:

1. Neck welling abscesses

This category of welling abscess, also called throat-pinching welling abscess, may grow at the side of the neck, in the submandibular region, or posterior to the ear. In his *Yang Ke Xin De (The Heart Attainment of External Medicine, Heart Attainment* hereinafter) in 1805 CE, Gao Bing-jun gave a good analysis of the generation of neck welling abscess when he says:

> In most cases, it arises from wind warmth and phlegm heat. When wind warmth ascends to attack, it inevitably stirs up liver wood. And with it, ministerial fire also becomes stirred. If ministerial fire counterflows upward, the phlegm heat in the spleen follows. The neck is on the route of the *shao yang* channel. When the evils which move along this channel come to the neck, they cause binding, thus producing welling abscesses.

At its onset, this type of welling abscess is as large as an egg. There is burning pain, but the overlying skin is normal in color. Seven to 10 days afterwards, the skin becomes red and the pain becomes unbearable. Later, purulence becomes mature, and the sore opens, giving off a yellow, sticky pus. By that time, the pain has diminished. After 10 more days, the sore may heal. In most cases, there are the generalized signs and symptoms of aversion to cold, fever, headache, a dry mouth, constipation, dark-colored urine, and a rapid pulse. These signs and symptoms worsen with the brewing of pus but get better with the draining of that pus.

2. Axillary welling abscesses

The Heart Attainment says:

> It grows in the armpit. There is no change in the color (of the overlying skin). The swelling has no distinct boundaries and no head... Cold and heat will appear before long. This disease arises as a result of blood stasis in the liver channel and qi congelation of the spleen. The swelling is difficult to disperse, and it produces pus in the end.

Treatment principles: Course the qi, move the blood, and resolve toxins. Since welling abscesses may occur in different places with different underlying disease causes, treatment plans should vary in accordance with the pattern.

Formula: *Da Zhui* (GV 14), *Tao Dao* (GV 13), *Qu Chi* (LI 11), *He Gu* (LI 4), *Qu Ze* (Per 3), and *Wei Zhong* (Bl 40)

Treatment method: Puncture *Qu Chi* (LI 11) and *He Gu* (LI 4) with a filiform needle with no needle retention. Prick the other points with a three-edged needle to let out a bit of blood.

Explanation of the formula: *Da Zhui* (GV 14) is the meeting point of the various yang channels. It is able to clear wind heat. *Tao Dao* (GV 13) is the meeting point of the governing vessel and the foot *tai yang*. It is a proven point specific for various heat patterns. It is able to resolve the exterior and quiet the spirit. *He Gu* (LI 4), the source point of the hand *yang ming*, is intended to course wind, rectify the qi and cool the blood. *Qu Chi* (LI 11) is the sea point of the hand *yang ming*. It is also able to move the qi and clear heat. *Qu Ze* (Per 3) and *Wei Zhong* (Bl 40) are indispensable in resolving toxins in many cases. When the above points are combined as a team, they are able to harmonize yin and yang, cool the blood and resolve toxins, transform stasis and scatter nodulation.

Other choices:

1. Prick *Da Zhui* (GV 14) and *Ling Tai* (GV 10), and then perform cupping over them. Puncture *He Gu* (LI 4) and *Qu Chi* (LI 11) using draining technique and not retaining the needle.

2. Moxa the sore over garlic till the pain disappears from the sore if there is any or till the patient feels pain if there is no pain in the sore before moxibustion.

3. Orally administer *Xian Fang Huo Ming Yin* (Immortal Formula for Quickening Life Drink). This is miraculous for various kinds of sores and is applicable in all stages. The formula is composed of: Squama Manitis Pentadactylis (*Chuan Shan Jia*), Radix Angelicae Dahuricae (*Bai Zhi*), Radix Ledebouriellae Divaricatae (*Fang Feng*), Resina Myrrhae (*Mo Yao*), Radix Glycyrrhizae (*Gan Cao*), Radix Rubrus Paeoniae Lactiflorae (*Chi Shao*), Extremitas Radicis Angelicae Sinensis (*Gui Wei*), Resina Olibani (*Ru Xiang*), Radix Trichosanthis Kirlowii (*Hua Fen*), Bulbus Fritillariae (*Bei Mu*), Flos Lonicerae Japonicae (*Jin Yin Hua*), Pericarpium Citri Reticulatae (*Chen Pi*), and Spina Gleditschiae Chinensis (*Zao Jiao Ci*). Boil and take with wine.

4. Orally administer *Tuo Li Xiao Du San* (Support the Interior & Disperse Toxins Powder). This formula is specific for sores which persist for a long time and refuse to open accompanied by stomach qi vacuity. It promotes the maturation of the pus, opens the sore, and generates new flesh. Its ingredients include Radix Panacis Ginseng (*Ren Shen*), Radix Ligustici Wallichii (*Chuan Xiong*), Radix Scutellariae Baicalensis (*Huang Qin*), Radix Angelicae Sinensis (*Dang Gui*), Rhizoma Atractylodis Macrocephalae (*Bai Zhu*), Sclerotium Poriae Cocos (*Fu Ling*), Flos Lonicerae Japonicae (*Jin Yin Hua*), Radix Angelicae Dahuricae (*Bai Zhi*), Radix Glycyrrhizae (*Gan Cao*), and Spina Gleditschiae Chinensis (*Zao Jiao Ci*).

Case histories:

In his *Wai Ke Fa Hui (An Aggrandisement to External Medicine, Aggrandisement* hereinafter), Xue Ji (1486-1558 CE) recorded two cases of welling abscesses. One patient suffered from hip welling abscess which was a hard swelling not yet purulent. At first, Xue moxaed the sore over garlic and administered two doses of *Xian Fang Huo Ming Yin*. The treatment relieved the pain. Then he prescribed *Tuo Li Xiao Du San* which facilitated development of pus. This was then followed by recuperation.

The other case had suffered from neck toxins with suppuration. Because the patient had dreaded puncturing, the toxins had spread to the chest where the sore was bright red. The patient had a rapid, slippery pulse. He looked fatigued and listless because the sore had made him sleepless for over a month and he had been unable to take in any food at all. Xue prescribed formulas composed of medicinals to support the interior for two months and the case was finally healed.

References:

In his *Shen Ying Jing (Divinely Responding Classic)*, the author, Liu Jin of the Ming dynasty, gave a prescription of needling *Jian Jing* (GB 21), pricking *Wei Zhong* (Bl 40) and *a shi* (points), and moxaing Riding the Bamboo Horse point. This last point is 1 *cun* bilateral to the point on the spine from which to the tip of the coccygeal bone is equal to the distance from the tip of the middle finger to the middle point of the wrist crease. From this classic downward, many Chinese have considered the Riding the Bamboo Horse point important for treating various kinds of sores.

In the *Lei Jing Tu Yi (An Illustrated Supplement to the Classified Collection of the Medical Classics, Illustrated Supplement* hereinafter) by the eminent scholar Zhang Jie-bin, there is a prescription of needling *Xin Shu* (Bl 15), *Wei Yang* (Bl 39), and Riding the Bamboo Horse point for welling abscess effusion on the back.

4
Flat Abscesses

There are a variety of flat abscesses named by their locations, for example, chest center flat abscesses, headed flat abscesses, lower abdominal flat abscesses, shoulder flat abscesses, celestial pillar (*i.e.*, back of the neck) flat abscesses, and forehead flat abscesses. Headed flat abscesses are those with one or more heads. Wang Ji (1463-1539 CE), a prolific author of medical works, gave a description of headed flat abscesses in his *Wai Ke Li Li (Illustration of the Theories of External Medicine)* saying:

> At first, this kind of flat abscesses consists of a growth of a white granule shaped like a millet grain but is itching and painful even by this time. The slightest touch will exacerbate this pain which may penetrate the heart... Three to four days later, its root becomes red and it extends rapidly with vigorous fever, slight thirst, and heat in the sore... This kind of flat abscesses has tens of white granules like pepper seeds over its top. In some cases, these granules may be as large as lotus seeds or cells of a wasp comb. (The sore) is purulent, but no pus issues out.

Disease causes, disease mechanisms

Such descriptions can be found in many other old medical classics. As to the disease causes and disease mechanisms, *The Origins* has an analysis of back flat abscesses which is typical of heading flat abscesses (in general). It says:

> All of the (viscera and bowel) transporting points of the bladder channel are on the back. When the viscera and bowels are disharmonious, the interstices are flung open. Then they are subject to wind cold which will frustrate the flow of blood. Thus binding and gathering arise resulting in swelling. If this swelling lies deep, this is a flat abscess; if it lies shallow, this is a welling abscess.

In sum, this condition is due to external aggression by wind cold or wind warmth at the same time that there is accumulated toxins in the viscera and bowels. After they invade, wind cold or wind warmth become depressed and then transform into fire heat. Internal toxins combine with this external fire heat thus putting the constructive and defensive out of order. As a result, binding and gathering arise which further deteriorates the circulation of the channel qi. In the end, a flat abscess develops.

In its initial stage, except for itching and pain, generalized signs and symptoms are seldom seen. But as the flat abscess enlarges, headache and no desire for food appear, and the pulse becomes rapid. Later, pain in the sore becomes more serious, and, with the growth of numerous pussy heads, fever arises. In the advanced stage, the swollen part decays and, with this, the generalized signs and symptoms abate.

Treatment based on pattern discrimination

In terms of its disease causes, there are two patterns of flat abscesses: vacuity and repletion. The typical vacuity pattern presents a sore which is flat and sunken with the overlying skin turning dark purple or a lusterless gray. It is slow in producing pus. In the case of yin vacuity with effulgent fire, there is scanty pus. In the case of vacuity of both qi and blood, the pus is a thin fluid of greenish gray color, and the patient has a white facial complexion and suffers from listlessness and somnolence.

Treatment principles: Course wind and clear heat in the early stage; disperse swelling and scatter nodulation to remove purulence in the later stage; and supplement the qi and blood in the advanced stage. Select pertinent points on the yang channels as the ruling points.

Formula: The ruling points: *Da Zhui* (GV 14), *Zhi Yang* (GV 9), *He Gu* (LI 4), and *Qu Chi* (LI 11). Auxiliary points: *Qu Ze* (Per 3) and *Wei Zhong* (Bl 40).

Treatment method: Needle all of these points using draining technique, except for *Qu Ze* (Per 3) and *Wei Zhong* (Bl 40) which should be pricked with a three-edged needle to bleed. Then moxa all of them.

Note: To supplement vacuity, one should also orally administer an appropriate medicinal formula.

Explanation of the formula: *Da Zhui* (GV14) is the meeting point of the various yang channels and, therefore, is able to diffuse and free the yang qi of the whole body. It also resolves the exterior and clears heat. *He Gu* (LI 4) is especially strong at rectifying the qi, while *Qu Chi* (LI11) is miraculously good at rectifying the blood. Their combination is able to rectify the qi and quicken the blood, course wind and clear heat. *Zhi Yang* (GV 9) is a point which is good at rectifying the qi and resolving dampness and heat. Pus is generated from blood and qi stasis, and to remove it, the qi mechanism should first be put right. *Qu Ze* (Per 3) and *Wei Zhong* (Bl 40) are miraculous at cooling the blood and resolving toxins.

Other choices: The above points can be moxaed directly with cones or indirectly over garlic. Moxibustion is good in the initial stage of this disease.

Case histories:

Gao Zhu-zhen suffered from a back flat abscess. This was a somber color, very hard, and made the whole back feel as heavy as if carrying a large stone. The patient's spirit was clouded. Mashed garlic was put over the sore. Over this was set a large cone of moxa. After twenty cones had been burned, the patient still did not have any sense of the cones burning. At this point, new mashed garlic was spread over the sore again and lighted mugwort was again spread over the garlic mash. This time too, the patient could not feel the burning. Then the cones were burned directly over the sore, and, after many cones were finished up, the patient began to have some sense of burning. The burning continued until pain was felt. Following moxibustion, a warming and supplementing formula of medicinals was administered. From the *Ming Yi Lei An (The Classified Case Histories from Eminent Physicians, Case Histories* hereinafter) by Jiang Guan (1503-1565 CE).

A male suffered from a back flat abscess. This consisted of a painful, red swelling which had spread over an area 1/3 of a meter in diameter. The threatening condition required a drastic attacking, *i.e.*, purging or precipitating, formula of medicinals. However, the pulse did not allow this. As an alternative, acupuncture was used instead. A bowlful of purple blood was let out by pricking the area of redness. In no time, the swelling and pain were relieved. Then *Shen Gong San* (Divinely Working Powder) and *Xian Fang Huo Ming Yin* (Immortal Formula for Quickening Life Drink) were prescribed. From *Xu Ming Yi Lei An (A Supplement to the Classified Case Histories from the Eminent Physicians)* by Wei Zhi-xiu (1722-1772 CE).

References:

There is one report of the treatment of welling and flat abscesses in which the treatment plan was to moxa each point in the formula above with 3-7 cones until the pain disappeared from the sore or pain was felt if there was no pain. Then the suppurative heads were pricked one by one. Finally, an appropriate paste was applied. For new or recent onset cases of flat abscesses, an average of 3 treatments effected a cure without fail. Lu Lin: *Zhong Yi Za Zhi (J. of C.M.)* 1982; (5):22.

There is another report of 25 cases of suppurative inflammation treated by bleeding therapy. The ruling point was *Wei Zhong* (Bl 40) which was pricked to let out 2-4ml of blood. *Da Zhui* (GV 14) and *Chi Ze* (Lu 5) were also pricked to let out 2ml of blood each. This treatment was given 1 time per week. Of the cases so treated, 17 were healed in 1 treatment, and the rest were cured by 2 treatments. Zhao Ming-ren: *Zhong Guo Zhen Jiu (Chin. Acu & Mox.)* 1983; (2):21.

5
Headless Flat Abscesses (Pyogenic Osteomyelitis & Arthritis)

There are a variety of headless flat abscesses. This discussion, however, is limited to the sticking to the bone flat abscesses *(fu gu ju)* and hip joint flat abscesses. (Sticking to the bone flat abscesses) may occur on any bone but occurs particularly often on the long bones of the limbs. Hip joint flat abscess refers to pyogenic arthritis of the hip joint. Because such festering sores first start deep within the muscle or within the bone, no abnormality is seen on the skin and even the patient may not notice anything wrong at their onset.

Sticking to the bone flat abscesses

In discussing flat abscesses, *The Spiritual Pivot* says:

> If vacuity evils penetrate deep into the body and cold and heat contend with one another, they may lodge in and stick to the internal for a long time. If cold prevails over heat, the bone becomes painful and the flesh withers. If heat prevails over cold, the flesh festers and the muscles putrefy, thus producing pus. This pus damages the bone. When the bone is damaged internally, there arises bone erosion.

What is spoken above as vacuity evil is usually liver-kidney insufficiency and qi and blood vacuity. This kind of vacuity is often the consequence of a major disease, for example, measles, cold damage, *i.e.*, typhoid, or scarlet fever. In addition, lesions of the bone, such as fracture, may also frequently be seen as the disease causes of this condition.

Treatment principles: Move stasis and free the flow of the network vessels, clear heat and transform dampness in the initial stage; drain pus when purulence is mature; and supplement and harmonize the qi and blood after the sore is open.

Prognosis: Poor if only needling and/or moxibustion are used.

Formula: *Guan Yuan* (CV 4), *He Gu* (LI 4), *San Li* (St 36), and local *a shi* points

Treatment method: Needle using draining technique. In the middle stages when purulence is mature, fire-needling may be used.

Explanation of the formula: *Guan Yuan* (CV 4) is able to supplement the source of the life qi, *i.e.*, the former heaven or prenatal qi, while *Zu San Li* (St 36) is a miraculous point for supplementing the postnatal or latter heaven qi, the source of generation and transformation. Combining these two harmonizes the viscera and bowels and the constructive and defensive in order to promote the maturation of suppuration and generation of new flesh.

Note: When faced with such cases, modern Chinese acupuncturists often recommend antibiotics and debridement as well as medicinal formulas.

Case histories:

A male suffered from a flat abscess deep to the bone while the overlying skin was normal. The pulse was rapid and somewhat slippery. This was a sticking to the bone flat abscess. When purulence was nearly mature, 6 doses of a formula for supplementing the interior to expel toxins were prescribed. Then the sore became painful and the pulse became slippery and rapid. When purulence was mature, pricking was performed and approximately 1 bowlful of pus was let out. A supplementing formula was further administered. Over 1 month of treatment achieved healing. From *Aggrandisement*.

A Mr. Yang, aged 32, came for treatment on Feb. 24, 1993. He complained of diffuse swelling around the posterior side of the elbow where a wound was found. Twenty days before, he had found a swelling and subsequently had undergone surgery to drain the pus. However, the operation revealed no suppuration. Two hours after the operation, he began to have a high fever and chills, and the swelling spread quickly downward along the posterior aspect of the forearm. Findings from examination included a bitter taste in the mouth, a purplish tongue body with slimy, yellow fur, a small amount of exudation from the wound, and a dark red color of the skin around the wound. Treatment consisted of debriding the wound, cake moxaing for 60 minutes directly over the wound, and the oral administration of a heat-clearing and toxin-resolving medicinal formula. After 2 treatments, some improvement was seen. Five treatments healed the sore.

6
Clove Sores (Pyogenic Infection or Malign Boils)

The Chinese word for clove sore literally means nail. This is because this type of sore is small, hard, and deep like a nail in the flesh. It is often seen on the face or the extremities, and it can have a variety of different names depending on its location and shape. Thus there are lip, whisker, cheek, and philtrum clove sores on the face; snake head and snake back clove sores on the hands and feet; and red thread, wool fiber, and hidden clove sores in other places.

Disease causes, disease mechanisms

Clove sores may be caused by various evils. If welling and flat abscesses or some wound are not treated properly, toxins may spread and flow through the channels and network vessels. This may cause clove sores. In addition, protracted emotional depression may produce effulgent heart fire which forces the qi and blood to counterflow. This, too, may lead to clove sores. *The Simple Questions* says, "(Pathological) changes caused by fine grain may produce major clove sores in the foot." From this statement, it is obvious that diet may also be a cause of clove sores.

Once a clove sore grows, its fire toxins may follow the channel, swiftly spreading here and there. Although it is small in size, its toxins are deadly, possibly and quickly leading to a critical condition and even endangering life itself. In treating a clove sore, the doctor should first be clear about which viscus and channel are involved and what is its root cause.

Treatment based on pattern discrimination

At its onset, a clove sore is but a small, pus-filled protuberance the size of a grain of millet with pain or itching. Gradually, the affected part becomes swollen and red, causing a burning pain with a deep, hard root embedded in the flesh. In severe cases, there are fever and chills and other generalized signs and symptoms. Later, all the signs and symptoms rapidly become serious and the head of the "nail" suppurates. At this time, thirst, constipation, yellowish urine, and a rapid pulse may appear. After the "nail" discharges its pus, the condition becomes less threatening.

In the course of its development, a clove sore may provoke yellow penetrating (*zou huang*), i.e., septicemia. In that case, the patient will suffer from vexation, agitation, clouded spirit, raving, distressed, rapid, dyspneic breathing, rib-side pain, etc.

There is a species of clove sore known as red thread clove sore. This is characterized by one or more red threads in the skin starting from the "nail" and extending with astonishing speed proximally like an arrow. The thread feels hard, possibly extending deep under the skin. In most cases, red thread clove sore is accompanied by serious generalized signs and symptoms.

Treatment principles: Clear heat and resolve toxins, disperse swelling and stop pain. In the later stages, support the interior and expel pus, cool and quicken blood.

Formula: *Ling Tai* (GV 10), *Shen Zhu* (GV 12), *Wei Zhong* (Bl 40), *Qu Chi* (LI 11), *He Gu* (LI 4), and *Xi Men* (Per 4)

Treatment method: Prick the first three points with a three-edged needle. Puncture the rest with a filiform needle using draining technique.

Explanation of the formula: *Ling Tai* (GV 10) is a proven effective point for sores. *Shen Zhu* (GV 12) is a point on the governing vessel. It is able to free the various channel qi and drain heat. *Xi Men* (Per 4) is the cleft point of the pericardium channel where qi and blood converge. As such, it is often used to treat emergency cases. Here, it is used to clear blood heat and check pain. As analyzed previously, the combination of *He Gu* (LI 4), *Qu Chi* (LI 11), and *Wei Zhong* (Bl 40) makes a good team for clearing heat and resolving toxins.

Modifications: If a clove sore is located on the upper limb, prick *Qu Ze* (Per 3) instead of *Wei Zhong* (Bl 40). One can also needle *Shen Men* (Ht 7) with a filiform needle. *Qu Ze* is equally as good at clearing heat toxins from the blood as *Wei Zhong*. *Shen Men* is the source point of the heart channel. *The Simple Questions* says, "The various categories of painful sores with itching are all ascribed to the heart." Therefore, performing drainage at *Shen Men* is able to cool heart heat so as to prevent toxins from attacking the heart. For red thread clove sore, needle *Chi Ze* (Lu 5) using draining technique, and prick the two ends of the thread, *Da Zhui* (GV 14), and the ten diffusing points (*Shi Xuan,* M-UE-1-5) to let out drops of blood.

Other choices:

1. Using a thick needle, insert it at *Shen Dao* (GV 11), thrusting it towards *Zhi Yang* (GV 9) beneath the skin (point-joining method) 1 time each day.

2. Get a piece of rush (Juncus Effusus) ready. Dip one end of it into oil, and then burn it. Put the flame for a minute over the end of the red thread of the clove sore and one will see that the thread becomes shortened a little. Then do this again to shorten the thread further. After several such maneuvers, the thread will be drawn back to the sore. Finally, do this at the same point as the first time to wind up the treatment.

Case history: In one report on an effective therapy for red thread clove sores, the treatment consisted of pricking the end of the red thread with a three-edged needle to let out drops of blood and then applying a disinfectant paste. Orally, a decoction of Rhizoma Paridis Polyphyllae (*Zao Xiu*) was prescribed. Of the cases studied, all were cured by an average of 2 treatments. Xing Yu-zhou: *He Nan Zhong Yi Za Zhi (Henan J. of C.M.)* 1985; 12 (2):127.

References:

The Orthodox Gathering says:

> If the sore first appears above the neck, one should prick to remove the malign blood to prevent the toxins from attacking inward. If it appears below the neck, one should moxa to thwart the (aggressive) tendency (of the toxins) in case they should invade good flesh. If the sore refuses to develop pus ... it is still necessary to insert medicinals (into the sore) and, internally, to administer some supplementing medicinals to expel (toxins).

The prescription in *The Divinely Responding Classic* is: "For clove sore in the face... moxa *He Gu* (LI 4), and for clove sore on the hand, moxa *Qu Chi* (LI 11)."

7
Cinnabar Toxins (Erysipelas)

This condition is also commonly known as red migratory wind. In addition, there are various other names for it. It is called sweeping fire if it happens on the lower limb, red migratory cinnabar if it happens in neonates, and internal cinnabar toxins if it happens on the trunk. If it happens on the face and head, a mild case is called embracing head fire cinnabar and a severe case is called massive head scourge. Cinnabar toxins is an acute infection characterized by sudden onset. Initially, there is aversion to cold, fever, headache, nausea, and retching and vomiting. Then it becomes a bright red, swollen spot with distinct boundaries. It extends rapidly, causing a burning pain.

Disease causes, disease mechanisms

The *Sheng Ji Zong Lu (The All-embracing Records of Imperial Benevolence)*, a brilliant work compiled in the Song dynasty under the guidance of the emperor, gives a concise explanation for its name and disease causes. It says:

> When heat toxin qi breaks out within the skin, if it is unable to drain out, it accumulates there into cinnabar toxins. Because the skin is red as if dabbed with cinnabar with yang qi hidden within, it is called cinnabar. Since heat qi is impetuous and swift, this condition is not fixed to one place. It may be as large as the palm. In severe cases, it may flow to all the four limbs. If it is not treated in a timely fashion, it will suppurate and fester. If this happens in the joint of a bone, it may cause loss of the limb. If the toxic qi enters the abdomen, it may kill the patient.

Treatment principles: Course wind and clear heat, cool blood and resolve toxins, disinhibit dampness

Formula: Ruling points: *Qu Chi* (LI 11), *He Gu* (LI 4), *Xue Hai* (Sp 10), *San Yin Jiao* (Sp 6), and *Di Ji* (Sp 8)

Modifications: Add *Yi Feng* (TB 17) for the pattern of wind heat. Add *Xing Jian* (Liv 2) for the pattern of damp heat. Add *Yin Ling Quan* (Sp 9) for the pattern of downpouring damp heat.

Treatment method: Needle using draining technique. *Qu Chi* (LI 11) may be pricked with a three-edged needle.

Explanation of the formula: *Qu Chi* (LI 11) and *He Gu* (LI 4) are both points on the *yang ming* channel, which is abundant in both qi and blood. Therefore, puncturing them may regulate the qi and the blood. In addition, these two points are able to eliminate wind heat from the head and face. *Xue Hai* (Sp 10), *San Yin Jiao* (Sp 6), and *Di Ji* (Sp 8) are all points on the spleen channel. Hence they are good at fortifying the spleen and transforming dampness. Moreover, *Xue Hai* and *San Yin Jiao* are both proven points specific for blood troubles. Therefore, they are able to cool the blood and remove toxins from it. There is a saying, "To treat wind, first treat the blood", since wind will die away of itself when blood is restored to normal. *Di Ji* (Sp 8) is a cleft point and, as such, it should be employed in emergency cases.

Other choices:

1. Prick *Yin Bai* (Sp 1), *Xue Hai* (Sp 10), and the *a shi* point. The *a shi* point is the bulging, purplish vein in the neighborhood of the sore.

2. Prick the *a shi* point and then perform cupping over it.

Case history: A 50 year old female complained of a recurrent, red, swollen spot on her left instep. She had been given antibiotics to no avail. I gave her several needling treatments but achieved little effect. Later, I used combined needling and moxibustion at 3-5 points chosen from the formula above in 1 treatment. Five treatments resulted in her recovery. On follow-up after 1 year, there was no relapse.

Reference: There is one report of 44 cases of cinnabar toxins treated by needling *Si Feng* (M-UE-9). Only the points on the same side as the sore were needled. If the sore grew bilaterally, the points were needled bilaterally. Of the 44 cases studied, 38 were completely healed; 4 showed marked effect; and 2 showed no effect. Wang Qing-yan: *Shan Xi Zhong Yi Za Zhi (Shanxi J. of C.M.)* 1986; 7(11): 528.

8
Scrofulous Lumps

There are different ways of naming scrofulous lumps in the old classics, and, therefore, we have a long list of different names for this disease in Chinese. In his work *Shou Shi Bao Yuan (Prolong Life by Protecting the Origin)*, Gong Ting-xian (1522-1619 CE) gave a summary of this disease by saying:

> Scrofulous lumps are the so-called bound nodes growing possibly in front of the ear down to the lower cheek and submandibular region or even possibly down to the supraclavicular fossa. Any such case is called a scrofulous lump. They may grow on the chest or the lateral side of the chest down to the free rib region. A case in this location is called saber. This is governed by the hand and foot *shao yang* channel. A small-sized lump standing alone is called a bound node. A number of lumps connected to each other are called strings, while those shaped long like clams are called sabers.

Disease causes, disease mechanisms

Scrofulous lumps are often impugned to emotional depression. If the liver qi becomes depressed and bound up, qi depression may transform into fire. Depression impairs the spleen's generation and transformation. This then produces phlegm turbidity internally. Where phlegm turbidity lodges, there arises binding or nodulation. Phlegm nodulation is the same as a scrofulous lump. Yin vacuity may also be an evil that produces scrofulous lumps. Yin vacuity generates internal fire, and this fire may boil fluids down to phlegm. This then settles in the channels and network vessels. If wind fire then attacks from outside, fire and phlegm combine, thus producing bound nodes.

Treatment principles: Level the liver and resolve depression, transform phlegm and soften the hard, or enrich yin and downbear fire

Formula: *Tian Jing* (TB 10), *Zu Lin Qi* (GB 41), and *Zhang Men* (Liv 13)

Modifications: Add *Yi Feng* (TB 17) for lumps on the back of the neck. Add *Da Ying* (St 5) for neck lumps. Add *Xing Jian* (Liv 2) for rib-side lumps. Add *Zhong Wan* (CV 12) in case of reduced food intake. And add *Tai Xi* (Ki 3) and *Gao Huang* (Bl 43) in case of yin vacuity.

Note: Select local points, points on the *shao yang* and *yang ming* channels, and proven points as the ruling ones.

Treatment method: Either needling or moxibustion is good.

Explanation of the formula: *Zhang Men* (Liv 13) is the alarm point of the liver channel and a meeting point of the foot *jue yin* and foot *shao yang* channels. As such, it is able to course the liver, fortify the spleen, and transform phlegm. *Tian Jing* (TB 10) is a proven effective point for scrofulous lumps. Besides, it is the sea point of the triple burner channel. Draining it is able to drain fire from the triple burner. Combining it with *Zu Lin Qi* (GB 41) has a proven effect for lumps.

Other choices:

1. Perform fire needling at the core of the lump if the sore has not yet opened.

2. Moxibustion. Ruling points: local *a shi* point(s), *Jian Jing* (GB 21), *Jian Shi* (Per 5), *Bai Lao* (M-HN-30) and *Luo Li* (around *Ge Shu*, Bl 17). Auxiliary points: *Jian Yu* (LI 15), *Qu Chi* (LI 11), *Tian Jing* (TB 10), *Guang Ming* (GB 37), and *Shou San Li* (LI 10).

Case history: The author has cured 22 cases of scrofula with moxibustion. As an example, a 17 year old female first came for treatment on July 29, 1991. Two years previously, she had found a swelling over her left collarbone. It was not painful and the skin was normal in color. When later it became very large, she was administered anti-tuberculosis medicines and had a surgical operation, but the wound refused to close. My prescription included cake-moxaing over the wound, applying *Sheng Ji San* (Generate Muscle, *i.e.,* Flesh Powder), and needling *San Li* (St 36). The reason why *Zu San Li* was needled with supplementing manipulation was that the patient exhibited vacuity of the qi and blood. Ten days of treatment and the patient was on the mend. Thirty more days and the case was cured.

References: Below is a collection of various treatments from sources:

1. Moxa *Ren Ying* (St 9) and *Wu Li* (LI 13) over garlic, 30 cones each.

2. Moxa *Zhang Men* (Liv 13), *Zu Lin Qi* (GB 41), *Zhi Gou* (TB 6), and *Yang Fu* (GB 38) 100 cones each. Moxa *Jian Jing* (GB 21) with the same number of cones as the years of age. And moxa the periphery of the lump with 7 cones.

3. Moxa *Jian Yu* (LI 15) with 7-9 cones, *Qu Chi* (LI 11), *Tian Chi* (Per 1), and *Tian Jing* (TB 10) with 14 cones, and *San Jian* (LI 3) with 21 cones.

4. Moxa at the hairline in the middle of the back of the neck with 7 cones. Effect appears instantly.

5. Moxibustion at the point 1 *cun* bilateral to and 2 *cun* above *Da Zhui* (GV 14) is specific for back of the neck and neck scrofulous lumps.

9
Bloated Cheeks (Mumps)

This disease is popularly known as massive head scourge and frog scourge. In the old classics, it is usually called sudden swelling behind the ear or cormorant scourge. It was possibly in the Ming dynasty that it acquired the name of bloated cheeks.

Disease causes, disease mechanisms

The Orthodox Gathering says:

> Bloated cheeks are generated by wind heat and damp phlegm. In many cases, it is an epidemic affliction as a result of a warm winter or untimely weather change.

If phlegm fire lodges in the *shao yang*, becomes depressed, and refuses to disperse, then the qi and blood may congest in the cheek, thus giving rise to swelling and fever and chills. The *shao yang* has an exterior/interior relationship with the *jue yin*. Since the foot *jue yin* encircles the genitals, toxic qi may follow the *jue yin* to invade the genitals and the groin. Therefore, bloated cheeks may be accompanied by testicular troubles.

Treatment principles: Course and dissipate wind heat, soften the hard and scatter nodulation

Formula: *Yi Feng* (TB 17), *Da Ying* (St 5), *Jia Che* (St 6), *Wai Guan* (TB 5), and *He Gu* (LI 4)

Treatment method: Either needling or moxibustion is OK. Use draining technique without retaining the needle if acupuncture is performed.

Modifications: Add *Da Zhui* (GV 14) or the tip of the ear, pricking to bleed, in case of fever. Add *Ye Men* (TB 2) and *Zhong Zhu* (TB 3) in severe cases. Add *Li Gou*, (Liv 5) and *Tai Chong* (Liv 3) in case of swollen testicles. Add *Zu Lin Qi* (GB 41) and *Feng Chi* (GB 20) in case of headache. Add *Ren Zhong* (GV 26, pricking),*Guan Chong* (TB 1), and *Zhong Chong* (Per 9, pricking) in case of reversal (previously translated as inversion) and clouded spirit.

Explanation of the formula: Since this disease is due to wind heat and toxins blocking the *shao yang* channel, selection of *Yi Feng* (TB 17), a meeting point of the hand and foot *shao yang*, is able to diffuse the *shao yang* channel qi to eliminate wind heat and toxins. Combining this point with points on the *yang ming*, *i.e.*, *Jia Che* (St 6) and *Da Ying* (St 5), is capable of dispersing congested qi and blood locally. *Wai Guan* (TB 5) resolves the exterior. As the source point of the hand *yang ming* channel, *He Gu* (LI 4) eliminates heat toxins and disperses swelling. This is because the *yang ming* traverses the cheek. When combined with *Jia Che*, these two act synergistically in clearing heat from the *yang ming* channel.

Other choices:

1. Moxa *Jiao Sun* (TB 20).

2. Puncture or press the auricular points: Cheek (MA), Parotid Gland (MA), Spirit Gate (MA-TF1), and Endocrine (MA-IC3).

Case histories:

A 7 year old male complained of fever, aversion to cold, no desire for food, and swollen cheeks. The patient was treated by moxaing *Jiao Sun* (TB 20) and administering *Chai Hu Ge Gen Tang* (Bupleurum & Pueraria Decoction). The next day, his fever abated and his swollen cheeks had improved a lot. This decoction is composed of: Radix Bupluri (*Chai Hu*), Radix Puerariae (*Ge Gen*), Radix Scutellariae Baicalensis (*Huang Qin*), Radix Platycodi Grandiflori (*Jie Geng*), Fructus Forsythiae Suspensae (*Lian Qiao*), Semen Arctii Lappae (*Niu Bang Zi*), and Gypsum Fibrosum (*Shi Gao*).

A 3 year old male complained of swelling of the left cheek accompanied by heat symptoms such as fever and a rapid pulse. The patient was treated by moxaing *Jiao Sun* (TB 20) and was cured.

References:

The Orthodox Gathering gives the following treatment strategy:

> At the initial stage when there is cold and heat, administer *Chai Hu Ge Gen Tang* (Bupleurum & Pueraria Decoction) to disperse it and externally apply *Ru Yi Jin Huang San* (Wish-fulfilling Golden Yellow Powder). If there is heat internally with a dry mouth and inhibited urination and defecation, disinhibit these with *Si Shun Qing Liang Yin* (Four Normalizations Clearing & Cooling Drink). After both the exterior and interior are resolved, if the swelling remains to be dispersed, purulence will invariably develop. Then administer *Tuo Li Xiao Du San* (Support the Interior & Disperse Toxins Powder). When the pus becomes mature, perform needling.

The ingredients of the first formula (*i.e.*, *Ru Yi Jin Huang San*) include: Radix Trichosanthis Kirlowii (*Hua Fen*), Cortex Phellodendri (*Huang Bai*), and Radix Et Rhizoma Rhei (*Da Huang*).

The second formula is composed of: Fructus Forsythiae Suspensae (*Lian Qiao*), Radix Paeoniae Lactiflorae (*Shao Yao*), Radix Et Rhizoma Notopterygii (*Qiang Huo*), Radix Ledebouriellae

Divaricatae (*Fang Feng*), Radix Angelicae Sinensis (*Dang Gui*), Fructus Gardeniae Jasminoidis (*Zhi Zi*), Radix Glycyrrhizae (*Gan Cao*), and Radix Et Rhizoma Rhei (*Da Huang*).

There is one report of 196 cases of mumps treated with burned rush (*deng xin jiu*). Of these cases, 51 were unilateral mumps and 145 were bilateral. The treatment method was to dip one end of a rush stalk in sesame oil, light it, and then swiftly touch the burning end to *Jiao Sun* (TB 20). This would cause a low popping sound to be heard. After that, *Da Zhui* (GV 14) was pricked to let out a bit of blood. One treatment was given every other day. Of the cases so treated, 183 cases were cured by 1 treatment, and 13 cases were cured by 2 treatments. Zhou Cong-ren: *Zhong Guo Zhen Jiu (Chin. Acu. & Mox.)* 1995; (2):15.

10
Sloughing Flat Abscesses (Thromboangitis Obliterans)

This disease was recognized in Chinese medicine as far back as *The Spiritual Pivot*. This classic says:

> It occurs on the toes and is named sloughing welling abscess. If it takes on a blackish red color, it will end in death without a remedy. If it is not, it is not fatal and is curable. If it does not yield (to treatment), cut it off promptly. Otherwise, it will cause death.

From *The Spiritual Pivot* on down, none of the other classics have neglected this topic. In his work, the *Ma Pei Zhi Wai Ke Yi An (Ma Pei-zhi's [Collection of] Case Histories of External Medicine)*, Ma Wen-zhi (1820-1903 CE) said:

> In the initial stage, the toes feel numb and cold. Later, they take on a purplish red color. Now the instep becomes swollen and hot, while the toes are still cold. The skin and flesh, the sinews and bones there become necrotic, and the joints gradually break open, issuing a foul fluid. The sinew is broken, and the flesh is shed.

What is even more lethal, this disease is progressive. As the author of the *Wai Ke Quan Sheng Ji (The Life-preserving Anthology of External Medicine)* published in 1740 CE says:

> Sloughing flat abscesses start in the toes and gradually advance to the knee, producing an unbearable pain. When the joints drop off one by one, death comes.

Disease causes, disease mechanisms

In most cases, this disease is originally ascribed to yang vacuity of the spleen and kidneys which are no longer able to warm or provide enough supplies of nourishment to the extremities. If then the body is exposed to cold damp evils, the qi and blood will become congealed and stagnated, producing obstruction to the flow of the channel qi and further aggravating the insufficient supplies of qi and blood. As a result, the skin and flesh become withered. There are also cases that may originally be ascribed to insufficiency of the liver and kidneys and to depletion of heart blood. In addition, emotional depression, heavy drinking, or external traumas may all also lead to sloughing flat abscesses.

Treatment principles: Course the channels and network vessels, move the qi and quicken the blood, dispel stasis and stop pain. Select local points as the ruling points and select points of the affected channels as the auxiliary ones.

Formula: *Tai Yuan* (Lu 9), *He Gu* (LI 4), *Chong Yang* (St 42), *San Yin Jiao* (Sp 9), *Xue Hai* (Sp 10), *Tai Xi* (Ki 3), and *Tai Chong* (Liv 3)

Treatment method: Needle using draining technique. It is better to combine needling with moxibustion. It is even better yet to also administer appropriate medicinals.

Explanation of the formula: *Tai Yuan* (Lu 9) is the grand meeting point of all the qi of the twelve channels and hence is able to rectify the qi. Furthermore, because the qi is the commander of the blood, it is able to normalize the flow of the blood vessels. *Xue Hai* (Sp 10) and *San Yin Jiao* (Sp 6) are used to fortify spleen yang and quicken the blood. The other four points are each the source point of a related channel. As such, they are able not only to cure local lesions but to supplement and boost the source qi in general.

Other choices:

1. Moxibustion: Ruling points: *Shan Zhong* (CV 17), *Ge Shu* (Bl 17), *Guan Yuan Shu* (Bl 26), *San Li* (St 36), *Chong Yang* (St 42), *San Yin Jiao* (Sp 6), and local *a shi* points. Auxiliary points: *Tai Yuan* (Lu 9), *Xue Hai* (Sp 10), *Yang Ling Quan* (GB 34), *Guan Yuan* (CV 4), *Tai Xi* (Ki 3), and *Fu Liu* (Ki 7). Moxibustion can be performed either with a moxa roll or cone directly or over garlic or ginger.

2. Prick with a three-edged needle the bulging veins at *Wei Zhong* (Bl 40), *Wei Yang* (Bl 39), and *Zu Lin Qi* (GB 41). Blood should be let out by pressing or cupping after the pricking.

References:

Xian Fang Huo Ming Yin (Immortal's Formula for Quickening Life Drink) is a prescription which is often preferred in combination with acumoxatherapy to expel toxins from within. This formula is composed of: Squama Manitis Pentadactylis (*Chuan Shan Jia*), Radix Trichosanthis Kirlowii (*Hua Fen*), Radix Glycyrrhizae (*Gan Cao*), Resina Olibani (*Ru Xiang*), Radix Angelicae Dahuricae (*Bai Zhi*), Radix Paeoniae Lactiflorae (*Shao Yao*), Bulbus Fritillariae (*Bei Mu*), Radix Ledebouriellae Divaricatae (*Fang Feng*), Resina Myrrhae (*Mo Yao*), Spina Gleditschiae Chinensis (*Zao Jiao Chi*), Extremitas Radicis Angelicae Sinensis (*Gui Wei*), Pericarpium Citri Reticulatae (*Chen Pi*), and Flos Lonicerae Japonicae (*Jin Yin Hua*).

There is one report of 181 cases of thromboangitis obliterans treated by needling. The ruling points were proven specific points, while the auxiliary points were selected based on the involved channel. If the focus was located on the lower limb, the ruling points were *Mai Gen* (N-BW-31), *Xue Hai* (Sp 10), and *Yin Bao* (Liv 9). The auxiliary points were *Yin Ling Quan* (Sp 9) and *Di Ji* (Sp 8) if the focus was located on the big toe. They were *San Li* (St 36) and *Feng Long* (St 40) if the focus was located on the second and third toes. They were *Yang Ling Quan* (GB 34) and *Xuan Zhong* (GB 39) if the focus was located on the fourth toe or the lateral aspect of the lower leg. And they were *Cheng Shan* (Bl 57) and *Kun Lun* (Bl 60) if the focus was located on the fifth toe or the posterior aspect of the lower leg. They were *Tai Xi* (Ki 3) if the focus was located on the underside of the foot.

If the disease focus was located on the upper limb, the ruling points were *Qu Chi* (LI 11), *Xi Men* (Per 4), and *Qing Ling* (Ht 2). The auxiliary point was *Shou San Li* (LI 10) if the focus was located on the thumb or forefinger. It was *Nei Guan* (Per 6) if the focus was located on the middle finger. It was *Tong Li* (Ht 5) if the focus was located on the small finger. It was *Wai Guan* (TB 5) if the focus was located on the ring finger. And it was *Da Ling* (Per 7) if the focus was located on the palm or forearm.

The needling manipulation stipulated that the practitioner should use the lifting and thrusting needling method after having obtained the needle sensation and then, coordinated with the patient, adjust the direction of the needle to make sure that the needle sensation reached the focus of the disease. After that, supplementing, draining, or neutral twirling technique were applied according to vacuity or repletion. Finally, the needles were withdrawn without being retained any longer, *i.e.*, without passive retention. One to 5 points were needled each treatment, 1 time each day or every other day. As an adjunct, pain-killers and antibiotics were prescribed in some cases. Of all the cases studied, 89 reported cure; 57 showed marked improvement; 31 were better; 4 had no effect. Zhang Huai-zhong: *Zhong Guo Zhen Jiu (Chin. Acu. & Mox..)* 1981; (3):10.

11
Breast Welling Abscess (Acute Mastitis)

This disease is characterized by breast swelling, pain, and burning heat accompanied by fever and chills and headache. In the old classics, it has many different names, such as suckling breast welling abscess, breast wind, and breast toxins. Setting aside that mastitis which has nothing to do with pregnancy or breast-feeding, there are two main categories of breast welling abscess: external and internal. Internal welling abscess refers to that arising during pregnancy, while external welling abscess is produced in the course of breast-feeding.

Disease causes, disease mechanisms

The disease causes of mastitis are fully expounded in the old medical classics. *The Orthodox Gathering* says:

> The breasts are under the administration of the *yang ming* channel of the stomach, while the nipples are ascribed to the *jue yin* channel of the liver. If the breast-feeding mother fails to nurture herself properly, stomach fluids will become turbid. Then this congested and stagnant fluid may transform into pus. There are also cases where worry and depression damage the liver and stagnant liver qi becomes bound, thus producing swelling.

The *Wai Ke Zheng Zhi Quan Shu (The All-embracing Book on the Patterns & Treatments of External Diseases*, *All-Embracing Book* hereinafter) published in 1740 CE says:

> There is a mass bound within the breast which is red, swollen, hot, and painful. If the mass is large, it is called welling abscess. If it is small, it is called a node. It is due to indignation, anger, depression, and mental stress or (eating) excessively rich flavors that lead to obstruction of the *jue yin* qi and blockage of the portals. (Finally, breast welling abscess) is produced by congestion and depression of the *yang ming* blood internally."

The Mirror says:

> Internal suckling breast welling abscess may happen in the sixth or seventh month of pregnancy when there is chest fullness and qi ascent. In the breast, there is binding and swelling with pain. If (the overlying skin) is red, exuberant heat is the cause. If it is not red, this is due to qi depression and effulgent fetal (qi). External suckling breast welling abscess is due to turbid qi of the liver and stomach and the hot saliva of the suckling baby. When the cool breath from the nose (of the baby) invades the

breast, it congeals and binds the hot breast milk, thus engendering swelling and pain and causing the woman to suffer from cold and heat, vexation and agitation, and thirst. There are cases where swelling and pain are generated (in the breast) without either pregnancy internally or breast-feeding externally. This is a trouble of the skin and flesh, and the breast sustains no injury. It is a product of congelation and binding of damp heat in the liver and stomach.

Treatment based on pattern discrimination

From the above classical explanations, it is easy to derive the following patterns:

1. Breast milk stasis & accumulation pattern: Underdevelopment or deformation of the breasts or excessive or overly thick breast milk may cause inhibition of the flow of breast milk. As a result, the network vessels of the breasts are blocked and the accumulated milk decays, eroding the breasts.

2. Liver depression & stomach heat pattern: Emotional disturbances, for example, frustration, worry, and indignation, may cause unsoothed liver qi, while eating excessively fatty meat and sweets may generate heat in the stomach. Unsoothed liver qi is the same as stagnation of the *jue yin* channel qi which governs the drainage of fluids. Therefore, the breast milk becomes sluggish and accumulates. If evil heat from the stomach steams this accumulated breast milk, it will putrefy it. This then results in the development of breast welling abscess.

3. External trauma pattern: Pressure or other forms of external force may damage the network vessels of the breast, thus causing obstruction of the flow of milk.

Further, treatment of mastitis is based on the stage of the disease.

1. The initial stage: There are nodes of various sizes within the breast with the skin normal in color or slightly red. The flow of the milk is inhibited. At this stage, there are often generalized signs and symptoms such as headache, toothache, chest oppression, nausea, torpid intake, no desire for food, yellow or slimy, yellow tongue fur, and a rapid, bowstring pulse.

Treatment principles: Clear heat and resolve depression, course and free the flow of the network vessels

Formula: *Jian Jing* (GB 21), *Shan Zhong* (CV 17), *Ru Gen* (St 18), *Shao Ze* (SI 1), *San Li* (St 36), *Tai Chong* (Liv 3), *He Gu* (LI 4), *Wai Guan* (TB 5), and *Zu Lin Qi* (GB 41)

Treatment method: Needle using draining technique. In puncturing *Jian Jing* (GB 21), insert the needle slanting towards the front. In puncturing *Shan Zhong* (CV17), insert the needle slanting downward and, after reaching the required depth, thrust the needle to the left and then the right. In puncturing *Ru Gen* (St 18), insert the needle slanting downward.

Breast Welling Abscess (Acute Mastitis)

Explanation of the formula: As mentioned above, the breast is located on the route of the foot *yang ming* channel, and the nipple is ascribed to the foot *jue yin* channel. This accounts for the selection of *Tai Chong* (Liv 3) and *San Li* (St 36) which courses the liver and resolves depression and downbears stomach fire. *Shan Zhong* (CV 17) is the sea of qi and hence is able to adjust the qi mechanism to free the flow of qi. When the flow of qi is freed, depression is resolved and the flow of milk is unblocked. Because the foot *shao yang* channel crosses the rib-side region, *Jian Jing* (GB 21) is selected to course and rectify the qi of the chest and the rib-side region. *Shao Ze* (SI 1) is a proven point specific for breast welling abscess. *He Gu* (LI 4) is able to clear *yang ming* heat, while *Wai Guan* (TB 5), which connects with the yang linking vessel, can resolve the exterior to treat fever and chills. *Zu Lin Qi* (GB 41) is able to diffuse and dissipate the qi and blood to resolve stagnation of the milk. Hence it is effective for distention and pain in the breast.

Other choices:

1. Using a long needle, puncture *Ge Shu* (Bl 17), pushing the needle towards *Shen Zhu* (GV 12) and retaining it for 60 minutes. This is actually a point-joining method.

2. Puncture *Jian Jing* (GB 21) unilaterally on the same side as the welling abscess, pushing the needle toward the affected breast.

3. Puncture *Jue Yin Shu* (Bl 14) on the same side as the sore, retaining the needle for 15 minutes.

4. Needle *Tai Chong* (Liv 3), *Liang Qiu* (St 34), and *San Li* (St 36), using draining technique.

5. Needle and then bleed *Da Ling* (Per 7).

6. Using a moxa roll or cones, moxa *Ru Gen* (St 18), *Shan Zhong* (CV 17), *Tian Jing* (GB 21), *Yu Ji* (Lu 10), *Guang Ming* (GB 37), *San Li* (St 36), and a number of local points. The moxaing may be carried out directly over the points or over garlic, ginger, or scallion. Another method is to puncture these points and burn mugwort on the heads of the needles while they are retained.

7. Apply a mash of scallion stalk, garlic, mashed loach, and potato or mixed fresh dandelion and cactus, dabbing it over the sore.

2. In the middle stage: The nodes are enlarged with burning pain, high fever, thirst for cold drinks, constipation, a red tongue, and a rapid, surging or rapid, slippery pulse. Later on, the swelling of the breast becomes more serious and the hard nodes become soft, demonstrating purulence.

Treatment principles: Clear heat and resolve toxins, free the flow of the breast milk and drain pus

Formula: *Ying Chuang* (St 16), *Tian Jing* (GB 21), *Nei Guan* (Per 6), *Xing Jian* (Liv 2), *San Li* (St 36), and *Wen Liu* (LI 17)

Modifications: In case of high fever and severe pain in the breast, add *Qu Chi* (LI 11), *Guan Chong* (TB 1), and *Da Zhui* (GV 14).

Treatment method: Needle using draining technique; see the above.

Explanation of the formula: As a cleft point, *Wen Liu* (LI 17) is intended to disperse severe swelling and relieve pain. Since now heat and toxins are effulgent, *Da Zhui* (GV 14) and *Qu Chi* (LI 11) become necessary, for these two are especially strong in eliminating heat and toxins. When the disease has advanced to this stage, all the three burners are involved. Therefore, the well point of the triple burner channel, *Guan Chong* (TB 1) should be used. It is able to break binding and congestion in all three burners.

Note: At this stage, it is often necessary to drain the pus by, for example, fire-needling. In addition, an appropriate formula of Chinese medicinals is often also necessary. Such a formula must contain large amounts of Radix Astragali Membranacei (*Huang Qi*) to support the internal to expel pus.

Other choices:

1. Prick *Da Zhui* (GV 14) to let out a drop of blood, and puncture *San Li* (St 36) and *Chong Yang* (St 42) with a filiform needle.

2. Rub the affected breast and moxa the local points before pus has developed. After suppuration, fire-needling should be used to open the sore and drain pus.

3. In the open stage: When the sore opens, generalized signs and symptoms like fever usually get better. However, if pus cannot flow freely, pain and swelling may remain as before.

Treatment principles: Continue clearing heat and resolving toxins, freeing the flow of the breast network vessels

Formula: *Shan Zhong* (CV 17), *Tian Jing* (GB 21), *Qu Chi* (LI 11), *Ru Gen* (St 18), *San Li* (St 36), and *Nei Ting* (St 44)

Treatment method: Same as above

Explanation of the formula: At the advanced stage, the focus of treatment should be on the *yang ming* channel to free the breast network vessels. Along with the other *yang ming* points, *Nei Ting* (St 44), the spring point, is particularly able to free the channels and quicken the network vessels.

Case history: A primipara, aged 28, came for treatment 20 days after delivery, complaining of swelling and pain in her right breast. The patient had previously been administered some medicinal formulas and hot compresses to no avail. The prescription was to rub the breast until it became red. One treatment healed the swelling.

Note: For breast welling abscesses at the initial stage, rubbing often works wonders because it may free the flow of the network vessels of the breast more effectively than many other modalities.

References:

In a report of 393 cases of acute mastitis treated by needling, the operation steps were to insert a needle to a depth of 0.5-0.8 *cun* at *Jian Jing* (GB 21), twirling it rapidly for 3-5 minutes to induce strong stimulation so that the needle sensation might reach the chest or the shoulder or even down to the arm. Then the needle was extracted without retaining it any longer. Of all the cases treated in this manner, 390 were cured, while 3 reported no effect. Of the successful cases, 220 were healed by 1-3 treatments; 59 by 4-6 treatments; 13 by 7-15 treatments; and 1 by more than 15 treatments. Gao Dian-kui: *Zhong Guo Zhen Jiu (Chin. Acu. & Mox.)* 1985; (5):13.

There is another report of 65 cases of acute mastitis treated by pinching. The practitioner pinched the skin along an oblique line from *Jue Yin Shu* (Bl 14) to *Ge Shu* (Bl 17) and from *Shen Zhu* (GV 12) to *Ling Tai* (GV 10) with their index and middle fingers 4-5 times till the skin became red. Of the cases so treated, 35 were cured; 12 had basic recovery; 7 showed effect; and 5 reported no improvement. Yan Cui-lan: *Zhong Xi Yi Jie He Za Zhi (J. of Integrated Chinese & Western Medicine)* 1989; 9 (11):692.

12
Shank Sore (Varicosity Syndrome)

This disease is also called skirt-hem sore, trouser-hem sore, or old festering leg. It refers to ulceration of a varicose vein, not just a varicose vein without ulceration. It also covers diabetic sores and ulcerations on the lower legs.

Disease causes, disease mechanisms

This disease is often ascribed to eating excessively acrid food and fatty meat which generates damp heat internally. Dampness tends to descend. When dampness downpours, it may obstruct the channels and the network vessels in the lower part of the body, thus producing shank sore. Shank sore may also be caused by vacuity of the spleen and stomach which causes the central qi to fall downward. Generally speaking, that occuring on the lateral aspect of the lower leg is a yang pattern due to gathered damp heat. Hence it is easy to treat. While that developing on the medial aspect is a yin pattern due to accumulated damp toxins and is, therefore, difficult to cure.

Treatment based on pattern discrimination

1. In the initial stage: There is a red, swollen patch with itching and pain on the lower 1/3 of the lower leg. If scratched, the sore may become suppurative.

Treatment principles: Clear heat and resolve toxins, disinhibit dampness and disperse swelling

Formula: *Yin Ling Quan* (Sp 9), *San Li* (St 36), local *a shi* points, and the sore itself

Treatment method: Needle the points using draining technique, and then moxa the sore. After that, apply *Qu Fu Sheng Ji San* (Dispel Rot & Generate Muscle Powder). This is composed of: Gypsum Fibrosum (*Shi Gao*), Borneolum (*Long Nao*), and Mercuric Oxide (*Hong Fen*). Or apply *Huang Bai San* (Phellodendron Powder) which is composed of Cortex Phellodendri (*Huang Bai*).

Explanation of the formula: Since *Yin Ling Quan* (Sp 9) is the sea point of the spleen channel, it fortifies the spleen and eliminates dampness. Dampness is usually caused by insufficiency of the spleen and can be eliminated by replenishing the spleen. *San Li* (St 36) is the sea point of the foot *yang ming*, a channel abundant in both qi and blood. As such, it is able to adjust and harmonize the qi and blood and to move the qi to relieve pain. Besides, it is a good point for banking up the righteous qi. The local *a shi* points are intended to free the network vessels, dispel decay, and generate the new. Moxaing the sore directly is proven effective for its healing since the circulation of blood is quickened once blood meets with heat.

2. In the advanced stage: The sore becomes sunken, constantly giving off rancid pus with the locally affected tissues turning blackish purple. The patient may suffer from distention and heaviness of the whole lower leg, generalized weakness, and fatigue. The tongue is pale with white, slimy fur, and the pulse is deep and fine.

Treatment principles: Supplement and boost the qi and blood, warm the channels and scatter cold

Formula: Moxa the sore and *Guan Yuan* (CV 4).

Case history: A retired worker, male, aged 76, complained of a festering sore on the medial aspect of both his right and left lower legs. The area of ulceration was about 5-6cm in diameter on the left leg and about 3-4cm in diameter on the right. The sores were dark in color. The surrounding areas were blackish purple. There were also some veins protruding around them. The treatment consisted of moxaing the sores over a medicated cake for 30 minutes and then applying *Di Gu Pi Fen* (Lycium Root Bark Powder). This is composed of: Cortex Radicis Lycii (*Di Gu Pi*). This was applied 1 time each day. One month of the treatment largely healed the sores.

References:

External application of medicinals also proves effective. The following quote is from *The Orthodox Gathering*:

> As for a sore of recent onset, one can apply *San Xiang Gao* (Three Fragrances Paste) or *Ru Xiang Gao* (Frankincense Paste) to heal it. To treat a sore of blackish purple color of long duration, one may apply *Jie Du Zi Jin Gao* (Resolve Toxins Purple Gold Paste). To treat an obstinate sore of years long with dark, black, sunken skin and flesh with a stinking smell, use *Wu Gong Jian* (Oil-processed Centipede) to eliminate wind toxins and transform stasis and decay.

The first formula is composed of: Calomelas (*Qing Fen*), Resina Olibani (*Ru Xiang*), and Resina Pini (*Song Xiang*). The ingredients in the second formula include: Resina Olibani (*Ru Xiang*), Resina Liquidambaris Taiwaniae (*Bai Jiao Xiang*), white wax (*Bai La*), Oleum Semenis Pruni Armeniacae (*Xing Ren You*), and Resina Pini (*Song Xiang*). The third formula is composed of: Cortex Radicis Tripterygii Hypoglauci (*Zi Jin Pi*), Flos Hibisci Mutabilis (*Fu Rong Hua*), uncooked Radix Rehmanniae (*Sheng Di*), and egg whites. As for the last formula, this paste is prepared from: Scolopendra Subspinipes (*Wu Gong*), Radix Glycyrrhizae (*Gan Cao*), Radix Angelicae Pubescentis (*Du Huo*), Radix Angelicae Dahuricae (*Bai Zhi*), and tung oil.

There is a report on the treatment of 40 cases of lower leg sores by means of needling and sunbathing. The ruling points needled were *San Li* (St 36), *Xue Hai* (Sp 10), *San Yin Jiao* (Sp 6), and *Shang Qiu* (Sp 5). The auxiliary points were 3-4 local points. At the local points, the needles were inserted towards the center of the sore. So-called sunbathing consisted of exposure of the sore in the sun for 15 minutes after debridement. Treatment was given 1 time each day with 5 days equalling 1 course. Between courses, there was an interval of 1-3 days. Thirty-four cases were healed and 6 showed marked improvement using this treatment. Lin Min-hua: *Zhong Guo Zhen Jiu (Chin. Acu. & Mox.)* 1987; 7(1): 51.

The author has treated 20 cases of lower leg sores. The treatment procedures included debridement, then moxaing the sore for 30-60 minutes, and finally applying *Di Gu Pi Fen* (Lycium Root Bark Powder), 1 treatment each day. Except for one case who discontinued the treatment for some unknown reason, all were healed.

13
Seeping Sap Sore (Eczema)

This disease is popularly known as yellow fluid sore. If it happens around the auricle, it is called ear-wrapping sore. If it happens around the umbilicus, it is called periumbilical sore. If it happens on the scrotum, it is called bauble wind. If it happens on the breast, it is called nipple wind. In fact, there are many more names for it. In the old classics, it is often called damp toxins sore.

Disease causes, disease mechanisms

The Orthodox Gathering gives a concise account of this disease's manifestations and disease causes, saying:

> Yellow fluid sore may occur on the head and face, around the ear, or on the back of the neck. A yellow fluid is suddenly generated. Then (the sore) breaks, issuing forth a sticky fluid. (The sore) spreads very fast, giving pain and itching. This is impugned to the sun beating and wind blowing and sudden aggression by damp heat. It may also be due to eating food which is damp and hot. There are (also) cases where wind is stirred up, generating fire (internally).

Treatment based on pattern discrimination

Clinically, two main patterns are seen concerning the design of the treatment plan:

1. Fulminant wind, dampness & heat pattern: This pattern amounts to acute eczema in modern medical terms and is characterized by exudation, acute itching, and redness of the affected skin. If wind is the predominant factor, the sore is liable to occur in the upper body or spread throughout the body with scanty exudation. If heat is prevalent, the affected skin is bright red, possibly with multiple pustules. If dampness is the predominant factor, there are multiple blisters with profuse exudation accompanied by chest oppression and torpid intake.

Treatment principles: Dispel wind, clear heat, and disinhibit dampness

Formula: Ruling points: *Da Zhui* (GV 14), *Qu Chi* (LI 11), *San Li* (St 36), *San Yin Jiao* (Sp 6), and *Feng Shi* (GB 31). Auxiliary points: *Yin Ling Quan* (Sp 9), *He Gu* (LI 4), *Zhong Wan* (CV 12), *Da Dun* (Liv 1), *Li Gou* (Liv 5), and *Zhong Ji* (CV 3). Use *He Gu* in case of prevalent wind.

Use *Zhong Wan* and *San Yin Jiao* in case of prevalent dampness. Prick *Da Dun* in case of predominant heat. And use *Zhong Ji* and *Li Gou* in case of dampness prevalent in the scrotum.

Treatment method: Needle using draining technique, retaining the needles for 2o-30 minutes 1 time each day.

2. Yin vacuity, dry blood & fulminant wind pattern:
This pattern describes the chronic, recurrent disease. The skin is dry and thickened with itching which is worse at night. The patient is usually emaciated, having a pale tongue and a fine, soggy pulse.

Treatment principles: Nourish the blood, dispel wind, and moisten dryness

Formula: Ruling points: *Qu Chi* (LI 11), *Xue Hai* (Sp 10), *Ge Shu* (Bl 17), and *Feng Men* (Bl 12)

Modifications: Add *Shen Men* (Ht 7) in case of vexation. Add *Feng Shi* (GB 31) in case of severe itching.

Treatment method: Needle using supplementing technique.

Other choices:

1. Moxa *Qu Chi* (LI 11), *Xue Hai* (Sp 10), and *a shi* points as the ruling points and *Da Zhui* (GV 14), *He Gu* (LI 4), *San Yin Jiao* (Sp 6), and *San Li* (St 36) as the auxiliary points. The *a shi* points are the center and the periphery of the sore. In addition, moxa all the places where there is itching.

2. Puncture or press the auricular points, Spirit Gate (MA-TF4), Heart (MA), Lung (MA-IC1), Liver (MA-SC5), Spleen (MA), and any corresponding, *i.e.*, tender points.

3. Perform cutaneous needling on the sore and parallel to the spine until there is slight bleeding.

Case history: A female, aged 52, had extensive eczema which had begun under her two breasts and was accompanied by unbearable itching. Because of this itching, she simply could not fall asleep at night. When she turned up at the clinic, her eczema had spread over almost her whole body, and she had lost confidence in recovery after having been treated for a long time without any effect. My treatment strategy was to clear heat and disinhibit dampness, quicken the blood and dispel wind. The treatment procedures included bleeding and cupping at *Ge Shu* (Bl 17) and *Fei Shu* (Bl 13), needling *Qu Chi* (LI 11), *Wai Guan* (TB 5), *He Gu* (LI 4), *San Li* (St 36), and *Feng Shi* (GB 31), and moxaing all the places that itched. After 10 days of treatment, the condition was under control. Then only combined needling and moxibustion was administered. Twenty days of treatment affected a cure.

14
Addictive Papules (Urticaria)

The term "addictive" implies that the itching is so unbearable that the patient cannot refrain from constantly scratching it.

Disease causes, disease mechanisms

There are several kinds of evils that may cause addictive papules. First of all, wind cold may be a culprit. If there is disharmony between the constructive and defensive, wind cold is liable to invade. Then wind cold evils settle in the skin and muscles. *The Origins* says, "If evil qi is depressed by wind cold which settles within the skin and flesh, then wind itching addictive papules will arise." The second possible disease cause is invading wind heat. Again *The Origins* says:

> People whose yang qi is vacuous in the exterior are likely to suffer from sweat draining. Sweating in wind results in wind qi contending in the muscles and flesh. (This wind) may then merge with heat qi. Thus arise papules.

Thirdly, a frail prenatal endowment, *i.e.*, a weak congenital constitution, eating a lot of fatty and fishy foods, *i.e.*, substances able to stir up wind and generate dry fire, or parasites in the stomach and intestines may all also be the causes of urticaria. And finally disharmony of the penetrating and controlling vessels and menstrual irregularity may lead to generation of wind and dryness which eventually results in addictive papules. These two vessels are closely related to blood, and dryness of blood is a direct cause of addictive papules. If one traces the origin of disharmony of these two vessels, one may find that emotional disturbances such as worry, preoccupation, and anxiety are responsible.

Treatment based on pattern discrimination

According to the above analysis, this disease is classified into the following five patterns:

1. Wind cold pattern: The patches are slightly red or pale and are liable to break out on exposed parts of the body. The condition becomes worse with exposure to wind and cold, but gets better when it obtains warmth. Therefore, it gets worse in winter and better in summer. The tongue body seems fat with white fur, while the pulse is floating and tight.

Treatment principles: Course wind and scatter cold, harmonize the constructive and defensive. Select pertinent points on the yang channels as the ruling points.

Formula: Ruling points: *Da Zhui* (GV 14), *He Gu* (LI 4), and *Feng Men* (Bl 12)

Modifications: Add *Qu Chi* (LI 11) and *Feng Chi* (GB 20) if the trouble is located above the lumbus. Add *Xue Hai* (Sp 10) and *San Yin Jiao* (Sp 6) if the trouble is located below the lumbus.

Treatment method: Needle using draining technique, retaining the needle for 30 minutes. *Da Zhui* (GV 14) and *Feng Men* (Bl 12) may be moxaed after being needled.

2. Wind heat pattern: The patches are red with burning heat and are liable to break out on the upper, covered part of the body. The patient may suffer from vexation and agitation. The condition becomes worse when affected by heat but relieved when it obtains coolness. The tongue is red with white or yellow fur, and the pulse is rapid and floating or slippery and floating.

Treatment principles: Course wind and clear heat, cool the blood and disperse papules. Treatment should be focused on the governing vessel, the foot *shao yang*, and the hand *yang ming* channels.

Formula: *Da Zhui* (GV 14), *Ge Shu* (Bl 17), and *Qu Chi* (LI 11)

Modifications: Add *He Gu* (LI 4) in case of severe fever and chills. Add *Shao Shang* (LI 1), pricking in case of swelling and sore throat.

Treatment method: Prick *Da Zhui* (GV 14) to let out blood and then perform cupping over it. Puncture *Ge Shu* (Bl 17) and *Qu Chi* (LI 11) with a filiform needle using draining technique.

3. Stomach & intestine damp heat pattern: This pattern is characterized by the complications of nausea, retching and vomiting, abdominal pain and distention, fatigue, torpid intake, constipation or diarrhea, a dry mouth and tongue, a red tongue with slimy, yellow fur, and a slippery, rapid pulse.

Treatment principles: Dispel wind, clear heat, and disinhibit dampness, free the bowels and clear heat. Select pertinent points on the *yang ming* channel as the ruling points.

Formula: *San Li* (St 36), *Tian Shu* (St 25), *Nei Guan* (Per 6), and *Zhong Wan* (CV 12)

Modifications: Add *Shen Que* (CV 8) or *Da Chang Shu* (Bl 25) in case of abdominal distention and diarrhea.

Treatment method: Needle using draining technique.

4. Qi & blood vacuity pattern: This pattern tends to be protracted and remittent. It is worse with taxation fatigue. The face is white and lusterless. There is fatigue, torpid intake, insomnia, heart palpitations, and shortness of breath. The tongue is pale, and the pulse is fine and weak.

Treatment principles: Dispel wind and secure the exterior, supplement the qi and nourish the blood. Select pertinent points on the foot *tai yang* and *yang ming* channels as the ruling points.

Formula: Ruling points: *Feng Men* (Bl 12), *Pi Shu* (Bl 20), *Qi Hui* (CV 6), and *San Li* (St 36). Auxiliary points: *Xue Hai* (Sp 10), *Shen Que* (CV 8), and *San Yin Jiao* (Sp 6)

Treatment method: Perform needling and then moxibustion or cupping. Drain *Xue Hai* (Sp 10) and *Feng Men* (Bl 12). Supplement the rest.

5. Penetrating & controlling vessel disharmony pattern: This pattern is characterized by its recurrent nature. It occurs 2-3 weeks before each menses and disappears with the stoppage of the menstrual flow. There may be complications of menstrual irregularity and painful menstruation. The tongue is dark purple, and the pulse is fine.

Treatment principles: Course the liver and resolve depression, harmonize and level the penetrating and controlling vessels. Select back transporting points and points on the liver channel as the ruling points.

Formula: Ruling points: *Gan Shu* (Bl 18), *Qi Men* (Liv 14), *Xue Hai* (Sp 10), and *Ge Shu* (Bl 17). Auxiliary points: *Guan Yuan* (CV 4), *San Yin Jiao* (Sp 6), *Xing Jian* (Liv 2), and *Qu Chi* (LI 11)

Treatment method: Needle all points using draining technique at *Qi Men* (Liv 14) and *Gan Shu* (Bl 18) and neutral manipulation, *i.e.*, neither supplementation nor drainage at the rest. Use additional moxibustion at *Guan Yuan* (CV 4) if there is cold congelation in the liver channel.

Other choices:

1. Moxa *Xue Hai* (Sp 10), *Ge Shu* (Bl 17), *Shen Que* (CV 8), and *Fei Shu* (Bl 13).

2. Perform cupping over *Shen Que* (CV 8) 3 times in succession in 1 treatment.

3. Bleed the vein posterior to the ear or *Fei Shu* (Bl 13).

4. Perform cutaneous needling at *Feng Chi* (GB 20), *Xue Hai* (Sp 10), and *Fei Shu* (Bl 13) till there is slight bleeding.

Case history: A 30 year old male had a history of nettle rash for over one year. He had been given hormones and some Chinese medicinals but no remedy had been able to prevent its recurrence. On examination, his lips, eyelids, backs of the hands, and upper limbs were all swollen and unbearably itching. His tongue was red with thick, slimy fur. His pulse was rapid and slippery. This was diagnosed as a wind heat pattern. The treatment strategy was to clear heat and disinhibit dampness, cool the blood and disperse papules. The treatment procedures included letting out 5ml of blood at *Fei Shu* (Bl 13) and needling *He Gu* (LI 4), *Wai Guan* (TB 5), *San Li* (St 36), and *San Yin Jiao* (Sp 6). On the night of the very first treatment, the swelling and itching disappeared. Five treatments and the patient was cured. One and a half years later, however, the patient had a mild relapse. The same treatment was given and no relapse has occurred since then.

References:

A Supplement says:

> To treat addictive papules, moxa *Qu Chi* (LI 11) bilaterally with the same number cones as the years of age. This is miraculously effective. To treat headache with addictive papules, moxa *Tian Chuang* (SI 16) with 7 cones.

The *Zhen Jiu Zi Sheng Jing (The Life-fostering Classic of Acupuncture & Moxibustion, Life-fostering* hereinafter) by Wang Zhi-zhong published in 1220 CE says:

> *Jian Yu* (LI 15) heals heat wind addictive papules. *Fu Tu* (St 32) heals addictive papules. *He Gu* (LI 4) and *Qu Chi* (LI 11) heal wind papules all over the body in either adults or children. And below, *Kun Lun* (Bl 60) heals wind papules.

In a report of 38 cases of urticaria treated by needling, the points needled were *Qu Chi* (LI 11), *Feng Chi* (GB 20), *San Li* (St 36), and *Xue Hai* (Sp 10). The ruling point was *Xue Hai* which was needled in all case. If the trouble was located above the lumbus, *Qu Chi* and *Feng Chi* were used in combination. If the trouble was located below the lumbus, *San Li* was used. Needle retention was required for 30 minutes with strong stimulation. Of the cases so treated, 36 were cured completely. Two cases reported cure but later relapsed. (No citation given)

15
Snake Cinnabar (Herpes Zoster)

This disease is also known as snake girdle or fire girdle cinnabar.

Disease causes, disease mechanisms

In most cases, liver qi depression and binding is responsible for this condition. Over time, depressed liver qi transforms into fire which then moves frenetically. This fire may find a conspirator in damp heat in the spleen and then spill over into the skin. There are also cases which are started by a combination of external toxins and internal damp fire. In addition, in old or weak people, this disease is often ascribed to blood vacuity with effulgent liver qi.

Treatment based on pattern discrimination

Based on its disease cause, snake cinnabar is classified as three patterns:

1. Effulgent liver channel fire pattern: The lesions have tight walls with red bases and there is a pricking pain. These are often accompanied by a bitter taste in the mouth, a dry throat, desire for chilled drinks, vexation and agitation, short voidings of scanty urine, constipation, a red tongue body with yellow or slimy, yellow fur, and a rapid, bowstring pulse.

Treatment principles: Course and drain the liver and gallbladder, cool the blood and resolve toxins. Select pertinent points on the foot *jue yin* and *shao yang* channels as the ruling points.

Formula: *Yang Ling Quan* (GB 34), *Xing Jian* (Liv 2), and *a shi* points

Treatment method: Needle using draining technique except on the *a shi* points which should be pricked.

Explanation of the formula: *Yang Ling Quan* (GB 34) is a meeting point of the liver and gallbladder channels, while *Xing Jian* (Liv 2) is the spring point of the foot *jue yin* channel. The spring point is ascribed to fire and fire is the child of the liver. When combined with *Yang Ling Quan*, draining *Xing Jian* courses the liver, resolves depression, and drains fire from the liver. Pricking the *a shi* points is in order to directly drain dampness and heat from the lesions.

2. Effulgent spleen channel damp heat pattern: The lesions are whitish yellow with loose walls which break easily. After breaking, the lesions erode, giving off an exudate or pus. In severe cases, necrosis and scarring are observable. The tongue is slightly red with slimy, white or yellow fur. The pulse is rapid and slippery.

Treatment principles: Fortify the spleen and disinhibit dampness, clear heat and resolve toxins. Select points on the foot *tai yin* and *yang ming* as the ruling points.

Formula: *Yin Ling Quan* (Sp 9), *San Yin Jiao* (Sp 6), *San Li* (St 36), and *a shi* points

Treatment method: Needle using draining technique except for the *a shi* points which should be pricked to bleed.

Explanation of the formula: *Yin Ling Quan* (Sp 9) is the sea point of the spleen channel and hence is able to fortify the spleen and disinhibit dampness. *San Yin Jiao* (Sp 6) is the meeting point of the three foot yin channels and has proven specifically effective for harmonizing the blood and clearing heat from the blood division. As the sea point of the stomach channel, *Zu San Li* (St 36) is known for its ability to support the righteous and dispel evils.

3. Blood stasis & qi stagnation pattern: This pattern, which is often seen in those who are old or weak, is characterized by severe pain persisting after the herpes lesions have disappeared, *i.e.*, post-herpetic neuralgia. The tongue is a dark color with white fur, and the pulse is thin and bowstring.

Treatment principles: Move qi and quicken the blood, warm the center and transform stasis

Treatment method: Select center-supplementing points such as *Zu San Li* (St 36) depending upon the particular pattern. Needle the local points and the points parallel to the spine, *i.e.*, the *Hua To Jia Ji* points. One may use a combined method of needling and moxibustion or cupping.

Other choices:

1. Moxa directly over and around the herpes lesions and then the points parallel to the spine associated with the nerve routes near the herpes. If using a moxa roll, moxibustion should be done for a comparatively long time. Or one should use a large number of cones.

2. Prick the herpes lesions and then perform cupping over them.

3. Perform cutaneous needling at the *a shi* points and the points parallel to the spine associated with the nerve routes near to the herpes until they bleed. Do this 1 time each day.

Case history: A 52 year old male complained of extensive, severely painful patches of lesions in the left rib-cage region. In addition, the patient suffered from reduced food intake and complete loss of sleep. Various kinds of analgesics had proven helpless for his pain. My treatment procedures included bleeding the herpes lesions and then cupping over them to let out more blood. This immediately relieved much of this patient's pain. After five days of treatment, the patient recovered.

References:

In a study, 30 cases of herpes zoster were reported to have been treated with fire-needling. The procedure was to thrust a red-hot needle quickly into each lesion and then quickly extract it. After that, gentian violet was applied. According to the report, 1 such treatment could relieve much of the pain. Three to 4 days afterwards the sore would be healed. All 30 cases were successes. Xu Chang-lou: *Jiang Su Zhong Yi Za Zhi (Jiangsu J. of C.M.)* 1989; (12):22.

The author has treated 52 cases of herpes zoster. Twenty of these had lesions in their rib-side region, and the rest had them in other parts of the body, including the neck, face, upper and lower limbs, and the hip. The results were 50 successes with 2 cases showing marked improvement. To treat such cases, I usually prick open each lesion. Then I prick a little more deeply several points in the area where the lesions are comparatively concentrated. And finally, I perform cupping over the pricked points to let out blood. This way a large amount of blood may be let out, but that does not matter. Experience has proven that frequently the larger the amount of blood let out, the better the effect. Many such patients have a bitter taste in the mouth. In such cases, I also needle *Yang Ling Quan* (GB 34) or *Qiu Xu* (GB 40). To prevent infection, I always apply gentian violet to the needled and pricked points.

There is another study of 100 cases of herpes zoster treated by needling. The points, which were all needled unilaterally on the same side as the lesions, were *He Gu* (LI 4), *Zhi Gou* (TB 6), and *Yang Ling Quan* (GB 34). In addition, encircling needling was applied. Encircling needling means to puncture several needles around the lesion, the number of inserted needles depending on the size of the lesion. The maximum number is 15 and the minimum is 4. In encircling needling, the needles are inserted slanting towards the center of the base of the lesion. Of the cases studied, 67 were cured; 11 reported marked improvement; 19 showed effect; and 3 had no response. The total effectiveness rate was 97%. Xu Jing-xia: *Shang Hai Zhen Jiu Za Zhi (Shanghai J. of Acu. & Mox.)* 1985; (3):6.

16
Oxhide Lichen (Neurodermatitis)

This disease may occur anywhere on the body, but the area most often affected is the neck. In the old classics, therefore, it is called lining-the-collar sore.

Disease causes, disease mechanisms

In terms of the disease cause, oxhide lichen is classified as two patterns:

1. Dampness mixed with wind heat pattern: This pattern is characterized by coalescing of the skin lesions into a patch and thickening and coarsening of the affected skin with red spots and scarring. The tongue is red with red spots on the tip, and the fur is yellow. There may be a bulging purple vein on the underside of the tongue. The pulse is rapid and bowstring.

2. Blood vacuity & wind dryness pattern: This pattern is often encountered in the elderly and weak. It is characterized by a whitish gray color of the skin in the affected area which also thickens and coarsens. There is also sloughing off of scales. This pattern is often accompanied by heart palpitations, insomnia, fatigue, and weakness. The tongue is pale with white fur, and the pulse is fine and weak.

Treatment principles: If the lesion is localized, only local treatment is required. For the dampness mixed with wind heat pattern, one should course wind, clear heat, and disinhibit dampness. For the blood vacuity and wind dryness pattern, one should nourish the blood, dispel wind, and moisten dryness.

Formula: *Fei Shu* (Bl 13), *Xin Shu* (Bl 15), *Ge Shu* (Bl 17), *Feng Shi* (GB 31), *Xue Hai* (Sp 10), *San Yin Jiao* (Sp 6), and the skin lesion

Modifications: Add *Gan Shu* (Bl 18) and *Yang Ling Quan* (GB 34) in case of liver depression transforming into fire. Add *Feng Men* (Bl 12) and *Pi Shu* (Bl 20) in case of wind heat mixed with dampness. Use *Feng Shi* (GB 31) and *Xue Hai* (Sp 10) as the ruling points in case of blood vacuity and wind dryness.

Treatment method: Needle all the points except the lesion, using lifting-thrusting method and rocking method to widen the needle holes so as to let out a bit of blood. Do not retain the needles.

The affected area can be treated by cutaneous needling followed by cupping or moxibustion over garlic.

Explanation of the formula: This disease is ascribed to the skin which is governed by the lungs. Therefore, *Fei Shu* (Bl 13) is selected to diffuse the lungs and resolve the exterior. Because the heart governs the blood and itching is always a manifestation of blood dryness or insufficiency, *Xin Shu* (Bl 15) is used to supplement and harmonize the blood. In addition, because this disease is often accompanied by heart vexation, *Xin Shu* should be selected to clear the heart and remove vexation. *Feng Shi* (GB 31), as its name suggests, *i.e.*, Wind Market, is able to drive out wind and hence to check itching. *Xue Hai* (Sp 10) and *San Yin Jiao* (Sp 6) work synergistically to harmonize the blood to remove the root of the disease.

Other choices:

1. Perform cutaneous needling on the lesion until it bleeds. It is better to increase the amount of bleeding by cupping after the needling. Treat 1 time every other day.

2. Moxa the lesion over a layer of mashed garlic at a number of points 1.5 *cun* apart from each other, 1 time every 10 days.

Case history: A 24 year old male complained of an extensive skin lesion behind his left ear and on the left lateral side of his head. There was severe itching of the lesion. Since there were no ostensible complications, only cutaneous needling was prescribed. It was performed on the affected skin until it seeped blood. Two treatments healed the case.

Reference: There is a report of 20 cases of neurodermatitis treated by cutaneous needling. For cases with extensive lesions, cupping was also used in addition to needling. Treatment was given 1 time every other day with 5 treatments equalling 1 course. Of the cases studied, 16 were completely healed; 3 showed marked improvement; and 1 had no effect. The effectiveness rate was 95%. The longest cases that were healed did not exceed 3 courses. Wang Ming-hua: *Shang Hai Zhong Yi Yao Za Zhi (Shanghai J. of C.M.)* 1985; 9(6):54.

17
Warts

Warts appear under a number of different names, in the old classics, for example, thousand day enduring sore, limp cow's hoof, and sinew-withering arrow. Infectious warts are called rat's breast.

Disease causes, disease mechanisms

In terms of modern Western medicine, all species of warts are ascribed to the same pathogen, viruses collectively know as human papilloma viruses or HPV. In Chinese medicine, however, individual analysis of the disease causes is necessary for individual cases, although warts often seem to differ from one another more by location rather than by nature. When discussing the cause and generation of limp cow's hoof warts, *i.e.*, plantar warts, *The Orthodox Gathering* says:

> When walking fast, the feet get hot. If one then puts them in water or they get caught in the wind, the qi may become stagnant and blood dry. Thus there will appear a binding or nodulation which is hard and tenacious. (As a result,) the constructive and defensive are obstructed and the swelling and pain gradually increase. The swelling is raised and protuberant, causing the foot difficulty in walking. Over time, (the warts) will break open giving off pus.

This is an account of the generation of warts on the foot *i.e.*, plantar warts, while the following passage, which is from *The Norms*, provides us with an instructive analysis of condyloma acuminata or perigenital warts:

> A male who indulged in fine grains and mellow wine suffered from hemafecia, bound stools, fright palpitations, and reduced sleep. Later, small-sized warts appeared around his anus shaped like rat's breasts...

Thus the author impugned this species of perigenital warts to diet. Therefore, since different kinds of warts have different causes, they must be treated in Chinese medicine by different prescriptions.

Treatment based on pattern discrimination

Flat warts

There are two sub-patterns of this condition: effulgent wind heat and liver depression/qi stagnation.

1. Effulgent wind heat pattern: The warts are slightly red and occasionally itch.

Treatment principles: Dispel wind and clear heat, rectify the blood and free the flow of the network vessels

Formula: *He Gu* (LI 4), *Qu Chi* (LI 11), *San Li* (St 36), *Feng Chi* (GB 20), *Xue Hai* (Sp 10), and the wart(s)

Treatment method: Needle using draining technique. One can needle the warts and then moxa them in addition.

Explanation of the formula: Since *Feng Chi* (GB 20) is the gate through which wind invades, it is often an indispensable point for dispelling wind and clearing heat. *Qu Chi* (LI 11) clears the lungs and resolves the exterior, while *Xue Hai* (Sp 10) communicates with the interior and harmonizes the blood. Combining these two can simultaneously resolve both the exterior and interior. *He Gu* (LI 4) is used to drain evil heat.

2. Liver depression & qi stagnation pattern: The warts are light brown in color and the patient suffers from irascibility and irritability.

Treatment principles: Course the liver and rectify the qi, quicken the blood and free the flow of the network vessels

Formula: *Xing Jian* (Liv 2), *Xia Xi* (GB 43), *Zhong Zhu* (TB 3), *Xue Hai* (Sp 10), and the wart(s)

Treatment method: Needle using draining technique. The wart(s) can be needled and then moxaed.

Explanation of the formula: *Xing Jian* (Liv 2) and *Xia Xi* (GB 43) course and drain the stagnant qi of the liver and gallbladder, while *Zhong Zhu* (TB 3) and *Xue Hai* (Sp 10) are able to quicken the qi and blood and free the flow of the channels and network vessels.

Note: In relation to both of these patterns, one may choose certain additional points in accordance with the channels that run through the wart(s). For instance, add *Si Bai* (St 2) and *Quan Liao* (SI

18) if the wart(s) grow on the face. Add *Shou San Li* (LI 10) if the wart(s) grow on the upper limb. And add *San Yin Jiao* (Sp 6) if the wart(s) grow on the lower limb.

Other choices:

1. Needle *Ying Xiang* (LI 20), *Si Bai* (St 2), *Yang Bai* (GB 14), and *Jia Che* (St 6) as the ruling points, and *He Gu* (LI 4), *Qu Chi* (LI 11), *San Li* (St 36), and *Nei Ting* (St 44) as the auxiliary points. Use 4-5 of these points in each treatment, retaining the needle for 10 minutes. Treat 1 time each day.

2. Puncture or press the auricular points Lung (MA-IC1), Subcortex (MA-AT1), Endocrine (MA-IC3), Occiput (MA), and any (other) responding or tender points. Use 3-4 points each treatment.

Reference: In a report on fire-needling treatment for verruca planae, the procedures were as follows: Get some sulphur powder ready. Heat the needle to red-hot over a fire and then quickly plunge it into the sulphur powder. Insert the neeedle into and extract it from the wart quickly. One treatment will effect a cure. Zhao Dong: *Si Chuan Zhong Yi (Sichuan C.M.)* 1989; 7(9):48.

Common Warts

If there is damp heat in the blood, the liver, which stores the blood, will become depressed. However, the cause and effect may also be reversed, *i.e.*, damp heat may arise from depression of the liver. In that case, because liver wood runs roughshod, it will rebel against lung metal. Then damp heat may lodge within the skin, developing into binding or nodulation.

Treatment principles: Level the liver and support the lungs, soften the hard and scatter nodulation

Formula: *Fei Shu* (Bl 13), *Qu Chi* (LI 11), *Jie Xi* (St 41), *Xing Jian* (Liv 2), *Xia Xi* (GB 43), and the "mother wart"

Treatment method: Needle all the points using draining technique. In the process of puncturing the mother wart, one should use lifting and thrusting method with force while twirling the needle. Then thrust the needle in different directions. And finally, widen the hole in the course of extracting the needle to let out a bit of blood.

Explanation of the formula: Since the lungs govern the skin and hair, *Fei Shu* (Bl 13) is intended to treat the root of the trouble. This is because warts are ascribed to the exterior. The lungs and the large intestine have an interior/exterior relationship. This fact accounts for the selection of *Qu Chi* (LI 11) which acts synergistically with *Fei Shu*. Because this species of wart is due to depressed damp heat which in turn involves the liver, *Xing Jian* (Liv 2), the spring point of the liver channel, and *Xia Xi* (GB 43), the spring point of the gallbladder channel, are selected in combination to course the liver and resolve depressed heat of the liver and gallbladder.

Other choices:

1. Insert a thick needle through the base of the mother wart. It is better to use a red-hot needle.

2. Directly moxa the head of the mother wart with small cones.

3. Apply a paste of mashed Fructus Bruceae Javanicae (*Ya Dan Zi*) on the warts.

Case history: An 18 year old male student had tens of warts on the back of his right hand, the largest being the size of a grain of maize. I moxaed the mother wart, *i.e.*, the biggest wart, with 3 cones so that it turned scorched black. Two days later, the wart discharged a bit of fluid. Ten days later, the wart dropped off, and half a month later, all the other warts disappeared.

Reference: In a report on 15 cases of common warts treated by needling, the treatment procedures were described as follows: After pinching the wart hard with one hand in order to reduce the pain needling will cause, the practitioner inserted a needle into the center of the wart down to its base to the depth of about 5 *fen* to induce the needle sensation. The needle was retained for 5 minutes and then twirled a little before extraction in order to cause a bit of bleeding. Of the cases studied, 13 reported complete cure after 1 treatment, while 2 were healed by 2-3 treatments. Gao Yun-ting: *Shang Hai Zhen Jiu Za Zhi (Shanghai J. of Acu. & Mox.)* 1988; 7(3):47.

Infectious soft warts

Treatment principles: Supplement the center, clear heat, and scatter nodulation

Formula: *Wai Guan* (TB 5), *Qu Chi* (LI 11), *San Li* (St 36), and the wart

Treatment method: Needle using supplementing technique at *San Li* (St 36) and draining technique at the other points and the wart.

Explanation of the formula: *San Li* (St 36) is chosen to fortify the central qi, transform dampness, and resolve heat. *Wai Guan* (TB 5) and *Qu Chi* (LI 11) are selected for the purpose of clearing heat and resolving toxins.

Other choices:

1. Break open the tip of the wart with a three-edged needle or a knife and squeeze out the cheese-like, semiliquid substance. If there are numerous warts, this operation can be done group by group at different times.

2. Moxa the wart(s) directly with cones.

Reference: The author has successfully treated 10 obstinate cases of infectious soft warts. The typical case is as follows: A 16 year old female complained of tens of infectious soft warts on her back, each the size of a soybean. The procedures included pricking the tips of the warts one by one, pressing out the whitish substance, and finally dabbing them with gentian violet. Three days later, all the warts were healed.

Plantar warts

Treatment method: Cut off the cutin to expose the base. Pinching the base with the left hand, puncture the base at three points forming a triangle to a depth of 5 *fen*. Twirl the needles to produce strong stimulation. Finally, press out a bit of blood after extraction of the needles. Treat 1 time each day with 3 treatments equalling 1 course.

Other choice: Electroacupuncture: Insert one needle into the mother wart connecting it to the anode pole, and then insert another needle into a local point on the channel where the wart is located, connecting it to the cathode pole. Retain the needles for 20 minutes. Treat 1 time each day.

Reference: Forty-four cases were reported to have been treated with block therapy at *Tai Xi* (Ki 3). Thirty-six were healed; 5 showed marked improvement; and 3 were failures. Wang Zhi-run: *Zhong Hua Hu Li Xue Za Zhi (Chin. Journal of Nursing)* 1985; 20(4):221.

Condyloma acuminata

This disease often occurs around the genitals or anus and sometimes in other parts of the body, for example, the armpit and popliteal fossa.

Treatment choices:

1. Moxa the warts.

2. Steam and wash with a solution of Radix Sophorae Flavesens (*Ku Shen*), Cortex Radicis Dictamni Dasycarpi (*Bai Xian Pi*), Alumen (*Ku Fan*), Radix Et Rhizoma Rhei (*Da Huang*), and Herba Senecionis Scandentis (*Qian Li Guang*), 2-3 times a day. Externally, apply combined *Qing Dai San* (Indigo Powder) and *Er Wei Bai Du San* (Two Flavors Vanquish Toxins Powder) mixed with sesame oil 3 times each day. The first formula is composed of Pulvis Indigonis (*Qing Dai*), Gypsum Fibrosum (*Shi Gao*), Talcum (*Hai Shi*), and Cortex Phellodendri (*Huang Bai*). The constituents of the second formula include, Realgar (*Xiong Huang*) and Alumen (*Fan*).

3. Perform fire-needling at the center and the periphery of the wart.

Case history: A 37 year old female came for treatment on Jan. 30, 1992 for condyloma acuminata. The lesion was as large as and shaped like a cock's comb and was located in the crease of her left labium majorum. The treatment procedures were as follows: After local sterilization and anesthetization, while the wart was fixed, it was cut with a red-hot scalpel lengthwise at its two sides and then removed. Three days after this operation, the wound was moxaed 2 times. Ten days later, it was healed.

18
Chicken's Eyes (Corns)

The Mirror says:

> Fleshy thorn disease is a result of bound up feet or walking in shoes that pinch. It causes difficult stepping and severe pain. This illness grows on the foot. Because it is shaped like a chicken's eye, it is popularly known as chicken's eye.

Treatment principles: Dispel stasis and generate the new, soften the hard and scatter nodulation

Treatment choices:

1. Insert one needle into the center of the clavus or corn down to its base and four needles at its sides obliquely towards the center of its base. Retain the needles for 20-30 minutes, during which time one should twirl the needles 1-2 times to strengthen stimulation. After extraction of the needles, press the needled points around their edges to let out a bit of blood. Treat 1 time every other day.

2. Perform fire-neeedling at the center of the clavus.

3. Moxa directly over the corn with a cone as large as the clavus after local anesthetization, 4-5 cones per treatment. After 5 days or so, the corn will wither and become easy to strip off. As a variation of this, one may first cut off the cutin to expose the base before moxaing. To facilitate the cutting, one may dip the corn in hot water for about 15 minutes to soften the cutin. As another variation, one may moxa over a layer of the Scolopendra Subspinipes (*Wu Gong*) and dark plum paste after cutting off the cutin. The paste is prepared as follows: Take 30 centipedes and 9 grams of dark plum. Grind them together into a fine powder. Soak this mixture in sesame oil in a glass container for 7-10 days. This paste can be replaced by a paste made from Fructus Bruceae Javanicae (*Ya Dan Zi*).

Case history: A 50 year old female complained of a corn on the sole of her left foot which had persisted for over two years. It had stubbornly recurred even though she had received various treatments, including surgical operation. I administered fire-needling and 1 treatment removed the corn completely.

Note: The curative effect is closely related with the depth of fire-needling. If it is deeper than necessary, the needling will cause great pain and possibly other side effects. However, if the needle fails to reach the base of the corn, it will not be able to make the clavus wither.

References:

In a report on 307 cases of clavus treated with moxibustion, the moxaing was performed directly over the clavus with cones until burning heat was felt beneath the base. All were healed. Xie Chang-ke: *Nei Mong Zhong Yi Yao Za Zhi (Inner Mongolia J. of C.M. & Medicinals)* 1990; (4):41.

In a report on 38 cases of clavus treated by fire-needling, the treatment procedures were described as follows: After local sterilization and acupuncture anesthesia in those cases overly sensitive to acupuncture, a red-hot needle was inserted right into the center of clavus down to the base until a sensation of emptiness was obtained around the tip of the needle. By then, a tiny amount of white fluid might have run out from the needle hole. Then the needle was immediately extracted without retention. The insertion of the red-hot needle was done at a moderate speed in order that there was time for the callus to be charred. If the red-hot needle cooled before it reached the base of the callus, then another red-hot needle was used instead to reach the desired depth. In this study, these 38 cases had a total of 49 chicken's eyes, of which 38 were stripped; 9 showed noticeable effect; and 2 had no response. Li Feng *et al: Zhong Guo Zhen Jiu (Chin. Acu. & Mox.)* 1984; 4(4):15.

19
Bedsores

Disease causes, disease mechanisms

Confinement to bed for a long time due to a major disease makes qi stagnation and blood stasis worse. This results in the skin and muscles losing their nourishment. Moreover, pressure on the parts in direct contact with the bed aggravates such stagnation of qi and blood stasis locally, thus producing decubitus ulcers or bedsores.

Treatment principles: Boost the qi and quicken the blood, course and free the channels and network vessels, harmonize the constructive and defensive

Formula: *San Li* (St 36), *Guan Yuan* (CV 4), *San Yin Jiao* (Sp 6), and *Pi Shu* (Bl 20)

Treatment method: Needle the above points. In addition, use the rounding-up needling method around the edges of the lesion. This refers to inserting several needles (transversely) around the sore.

Explanation of the formula: *Guan Yuan* (CV 4) is intended to supplement the original yang or the source qi. *San Li* (St 36) is able to boost the righteous. Combined with it, *Pi Shu* (Bl 20) fortifies the spleen and stomach to support the postnatal source qi. *San Yin Jiao* (Sp 6) is a particularly good point for quickening the blood and transforming stasis. When these points are combined together, their effect of boosting the qi and quickening the blood, freeing the channels and harmonizing the constructive and defensive is marked.

Note: To be effective, any therapy must be accompanied by careful attendance to the patient. Clinical experience shows that needling these points serves only as an aid in some cases, and local treatment should be given priority. Moxibustion is the best choice for local treatment. When red macules first appear, *i.e.*, before the lesions have ulcerated, moxibustion over the affected area easily effects healing. For severe cases of decubitus ulcers, one may needle around the affected part(s) and then moxa them. In addition, some appropriate Western medicine or Chinese medicinal paste can be applied.

Case histories:

Bedsores seem to be an ignored area in the Chinese acumoxa literature, and there is a lack of classical cites supporting acupuncture and moxibustion's efficacy in the treatment of this condition. In my 20 years of practice, I have treated scores of such cases and am a witness to the miraculous effectiveness of this therapy.

A 52 year old male had a bone fracture from a traffic accident. As a result of his long bed-ridden condition, he suffered from bedsores in the sacrococcygeal region. Merely moxaing the affected part 10 times healed the lesion without employing other therapies as aids.

A 32 year old female was a victim of uremia due to kidney tuberculosis. As a result of overly long confinement to bed, maltreatment, and ill attendance, the patient suffered from a terrible bedsore which had eroded her sacrococcygeal region to such a terrible extent that there was no skin and flesh left on the larger part of the region, some bones being exposed. The patient had a pale face, spirit abstraction, and extreme weakness. Her pattern was diagnosed as kidney yin and yang dual debility. The treament included needling, moxibustion, and medication. Fifty days of such a treatment healed the sore. The needling and moxibustion method were as instructed above. The medication included oral administration of *Jin Gui Shen Qi Wan* (Gold Cabinet Kidney Qi Pills) and *Shi Quan Da Bu Wan* (Ten Completely & Greatly Supplementing Pills) and external application of *Di Gu Pi Fen* (Lycium Root Bark Powder).

The first formula is composed of uncooked Radix Rehmanniae (*Sheng Di*), Radix Dioscoreae Oppositae (*Shan Yao*), Fructus Corni Officinalis (*Shan Zhu Yu*), Rhizoma Alismatis (*Ze Xie*), Sclerotium Poriae Cocos (*Fu Ling*), Ramulus Cinnamomi Cassiae (*Gui Zhi*), blast-fried Radix Lateralis Praeparatus Aconiti Carmichaeli (*Pao Fu Zi*), and Cortex Radicis Moutan (*Dan Pi*).

The second formula is composed of the following ingredients: Radix Panacis Ginseng (*Ren Shen*), Cortex Cinnamomi Cassiae (*Rou Gui*), Radix Ligustici Wallichii (*Chuan Xiong*), Sclerotium Poriae Cocos (*Fu Ling*), Radix Rehmanniae (*Di Huang*), Rhizoma Atrctylodis Macrocephalae (*Bai Zhu*), Radix Glycyrrhizae (*Gan Cao*), Radix Angelicae Sinensis (*Dang Gui*), Radix Astragali Membranacei (*Huang Qi*), and Radix Paeoniae Lactiflorae (*Shao Yao*).

The powder for the third formula is prepared from Cortex Radicis Lycii Chinensis (*Di Gu Pi*), Radix Glycyrrhizae (*Gan Cao*), Radix Panacis Ginseng (*Ren Sheng*), Radix Bupleuri (*Chai Hu*), and Cornu Antelopis Saiga-tatarici (*Ling Yang Jiao*). One can substitute Cornu Caprae (*Shan Yang Jiao*) or goat horn for this endangered species.

Reference: There is a report of 50 cases of decubitus ulcers treated with mugwort fumigation followed by moxibustion. All the cases were cured. Mild cases healed in 1-2 days, and severe cases with ulceration of various degrees healed in 3-15 days. The mugwort fumigation was done as follows: A certain amount of Folium Artemisiae Argyii (*Ai Ye*) was placed in a container which had an opening to let smoke out when the mugwort was being burned. The sore which had undergone debridement was positioned right over this rising smoke. This fumigation was continued until a thin, yellow layer of mugwort oil formed over the lesion. Yao Yu-fang: *An Hui Zhong Yi Xue Yuan Xue Bao (Academic Journal of Anhui C.M. Institute)* 1989; 8(3):587.

20
Drinker's Nose (Acne Rosacea)

Disease causes, disease mechanisms

If heat accumulates in the lung channel, this heat may be depressed and contend with the blood. When hot blood enters the portal of the lungs, *i.e.*, the nose, it tinges the nose a red color. There are also cases where there is damp heat in the stomach and intestines fuming the lungs. When this damp heat follows the lung channel up into the nose, it may become depressed within the skin if it meets with external wind cold. Then it renders the nose red. Damp heat in the stomach and intestines may be produced by eating too much acrid food or drinking too much alcohol. *The Mirror* says:

> This disease starts in the tip and lateral sides of the nose. If stomach fire fumes the lungs and is bound up externally by wind cold, there will be blood stasis. As a result, drinker's nose appears.

Treatment based on pattern discrimination

There are two patterns of this disease based on its disease causes.

1. Heat accumulation pattern

A. Lung/stomach heat accumulation pattern: The affected skin gradually becomes red with an oily, slimy luster. The red patch becomes worse when affected by heat or emotional agitation. There is itching accompanied by thirst and a desire for water. The tongue is red with yellow fur, and the pulse is rapid.

B. Stasis mixed with damp heat pattern: The affected skin is dark red with a small number of blood threads, *i.e.*, visible vessels, and papules or pustules. The stools are dry with short voidings of scanty urine. The tongue fur is yellow and slimy, and the pulse is rapid and slippery.

Treatment principles: Clear accumulated heat from the lungs and stomach, quicken the blood and transform stasis, cool the blood and drain heat

Formula: Ruling points: *Yin Tang* (M-HN-3), *Su Liao* (GV 25), *Ying Xiang* (LI 20), *Di Cang* (St

4), *Cheng Jiang* (CV 24), and *Quan Liao* (SI 18). Auxiliary points: *He Liao* (LI 19), *Ju Liao* (St 3), *Da Ying* (St 5), *He Gu* (LI 4), and *Qu Chi* (LI 11).

Treatment method: Needle a group of 3-5 points chosen from the above 2 times each week, using the points by turns. Insert the needles to a shallow depth and retain them for 15 minutes. Insert the needles slowly but extract them quickly. Press the needle holes after extraction of the needles to promote the discharge of drops of blood.

Explanation of the formula: This formula gives priority to the yang and especially to the *yang ming* channels which are abundant in blood and qi. Accumulated heat is a yang evil and it can be most effectively drained through the yang channels. In addition, bleeding is a good aid in clearing heat and dissipating depression. It should be noticed that, although there is heat in the lungs which needs draining, points on the hand *yang ming* are chosen. This is because the large intestine and lungs are a team having an exterior/interior relationship.

2. Blood stasis & retained toxins pattern: The nose is dark red and its skin gradually thickens. There is the possible growth of tumor-like polyps, and there is slight itching. The tongue is dark red, possibly with static spots, and the pulse is bowstring and choppy.

Treatment principles: Quicken the blood, transform stasis, and free the flow of the network vessels

Formula: *Su Liao* (GV 25), *He Gu* (LI 4), and the prominent veins around the nose

Treatment method: Puncture *He Gu* (LI 4) with a filiform needle using draining technique, retaining the needle for 15 minutes. Prick the other points to let out a bit of blood.

Explanation of the formula: *Su Liao* (GV 25), which is located at the tip of the nose, is able not only to harmonize the qi of the governing vessel but free the qi and blood around the nose. Its action is strengthened by *He Gu* (LI 4).

Other choices:

1. Prick *Su Liao* (GV 25) 2 times per week. Needle *Fei Shu* (Bl 13) and *Ge Shu* (Bl 17) using draining technique 1 time each day.

2. Gently beat the affected part with a cutaneous needle 1 time each day.

3. Puncture or press the auricular points Nose (MA-T1), Lung (MA-IC1), Endocrine (MA-IC3), and Adrenal (MA).

4. Apply a paste prepared from powdered Radix Et Rhizoma Rhei (*Da Huang*) and Sulphur (*Liu Huang*) mixed with cold water 1 time each day.

Case history: A woman more than 50 years old had red patches all over her nose with pustules and colored patterns over her cheeks. The treatment plan was to free the flow of the network vessels locally and to eliminate heat toxins. *Su Liao* (GV 25) was chosen. After pricking it 2 times, the patches obviously became lighter in color and 5 treatments healed the patches.

Reference: In a report on 37 cases of drinker's nose treated with needling, the treatment procedures included pricking with a fine needle 20 points per square centimeter on the affected region of the nose to let out a bit of blood. Then *Yin Tang* (M-HN-3) and *Ying Xiang* (LI 20) were needled. Treatment was given 1 time each day with 7 days equalling 1 course. The results were 26 successes; 8 cases showed effect; but 2 cases were failures. This study showed that the more protracted the condition, the less likely it could be healed. The two failures were both cases of enduring pachyderma. (No cite given)

21
Frozen Sore (Frostbite & Hypothermia)

Disease causes, disease mechanisms

The Origins gives an analysis of the causes of this lesion by saying:

> Exposed to wind, snow, and cold toxins during the three months of cold winter, the skin and flesh may be damaged with the blood and qi becoming congested and impeded. As a result, a frozen sore is produced which takes on a brilliant red color with swelling and pain.

This lesion has something to do with one's bodily physique. Those who cannot endure cold are liable to contract it. Furthermore, improper treatment is also a factor responsible for its development. *The Mirror* says:

> Suppose one is frostbitten. If one immediately approaches a heat (source), enters a warm room, gets heated by a fire, or washes with hot water, this will unavoidably make the flesh die and damage the form. In a mild case, the flesh decays and rots, while in a severe case, bone desertion will arise affecting the sinews.

In most cases, frostbite is localized, the lesion only affecting the extremities. However, long exposure to severe chill may cause a critical generalized condition.

Treatment based on pattern discrimination

1. Generalized "frostbite" (*i.e.*, life-threatening hypothermia): Due to cold penetrating deep throughout the body, at first the fingers of the hands and toes of the feet become painful and then become numb. Next, possible loss of consciousness occurs with dilated pupils of the eyes, rigidity of the body, and faint breathing. The pulse is very fine and weak, on the verge of expiry.

Treatment principles: Recover yang and stem counterflow, resolve freezing and bring life back

Formula: *Nei Guan* (Per 6), *Ren Zhong* (GV 26), *Shen Que* (CV 8), *Guan Yuan* (CV 4), *Qi Hai* (CV 6), and *Yong Quan* (Ki 1)

Treatment method: Needle the first two points with strong stimulation, using draining technique. Moxa the next three points for a long time till the patient regains consciousness. Then needle and later moxa the last point.

Explanation of the formula: *Nei Guan* (Per 6) directly communicates with the heart, and *Ren Zhong* (GV 26) is a specific point for emergency cases because it is able to arouse the brain and open the portals. Needling them recovers the spirit. The points *Shen Que* (CV 8), *Guan Yuan* (CV 4), and *Qi Hai* (CV 6) are miraculous for restoring the source qi, and, when they are used in combination and more particularly are moxaed, they can send heat qi or yang qi straight into the Cinnabar Field (*Dan Tian*) where life's qi is generated. *Yong Quan* (Ki 1) is the well point of the kidney channel, a channel ascribed to true winter/water, so it is not only able to resuscitate life but is most appropriate for problems caused by winter/water. Moreover, the kidneys are the viscera where true yang or true fire is stored, and they can be best fortified by their spring well point.

2. Localized frostbite: The lesion is usually confined to the tips of the limbs or other protruding parts like the tip of the nose and cheeks.

Treatment principles: Warm the channels and quicken the blood

Treatment choices:

1. Moxa the affected part. It is better to do this over Cortex Phellodendri (*Huang Bai*), Radix Et Rhizoma Rhei (*Da Huang*), Fructus Crataegi (*Shan Zha*), ginger, or a mixture of powdered Mirabilitum (*Mang Xiao*) and Cortex Phellodendri (*Huang Bai*).

2. Combined needling & moxibustion: Insert needles around the affected area at points one *cun* apart from each other. Then light mugwort on the heads of the needles while they are retained. One may additionally needle *San Li* (St 36), *Ming Men* (GV 4), *Pi Shu* (Bl 20), and *Shen Shu* (Bl 23) using draining technique. If the affected skin has already turned blackish or purple, one may prick the ten diffusing points (*Shi Xuan*, M-UE-1-5).

Note: For either of the above patterns, one may orally administer *Ren Shen Yang Rong Tang* (Ginseng Nourish the Constructive Decoction). This is composed of uncooked Radix Rehmannia (*Sheng Di*), Radix Paeoniae Lactiflorae (*Shao Yao*), Radix Angelicae Sinensis (*Dang Gui*), Rhizoma Atractylodis Macrocephalae (*Bai Zhu*), Sclerotium Poriae Cocos (*Fu Ling*), Radix Glycyrrhizae (*Gan Cao*), Cortex Cinnamomi Cassiae (*Gui Xin*), Radix Astragalus Membranacei (*Huang Qi*), Pericarpium Citri Reticulatae (*Chen Pi*), Radix Polygalae Tenuifoliae (*Yuan Zhi*), Rhizoma Gingiberis (*Jiang*), and Fructus Zizyphi Jujubae (*Da Zao*).

Case history: The author once got frostbitten on the toes of her feet while travelling. These became swollen and painful. Moxibustion with a moxa roll 2 times healed the sore.

References:

Because acupuncture and moxibustion can quicken the blood and transform stasis, recover yang and restore consciousness, Chinese practitioners often prefer it for treating forstbite or generalized frostbite, *i.e.*, hypothermia. Therefore, there is a wealth of reports on the treatment of frostbite with acupuncture and moxibustion since the liberation of the mainland in 1949.

There is one report of 1,000 cases treated with needling. Puncturing was performed in the affected local areas. One to 4 points were selected, the number depending on the size of the sore. After insertion, lifting and thrusting method was performed while the needle was twirled. The needle was not retained. After extraction, the practitioner might gently rub the affected part and press out a bit of blood from the needled holes. Of the cases so treated, 922 were healed, of which 825 required only 1 treatment. Forty-seven improved, and 31 showed no effect. The total effectiveness rate was 96%. Zhang Jun-tao: *Zhong Guo Zhen Jiu (Chin. Acu. & Mox.)* 1986; 6(6):54.

There is another report of 79 cases treated by directly moxaing the affected parts. Seventy-two of these cases were healed. Tian Pei-lin: *Zhong Guo Zhen Jiu (Chin. Acu. & Mox.)* 1982; 46(6):5.

There is yet another report of 70 cases treated with a paste made from Mirabiltium (*Mang Xiao*). All were healed. Wu Shi-chang: *Zhong Yi Za Zhi (J. of C.M.)* 1984; (2):75.

22
Pricking Powder (Acne Vulgaris)

Disease causes, disease mechanisms

The Simple Questions says, "Sweating in a draft while working provides a chance for cold to invade, and hence gives rise to pricks." Wang Bin (710-804 CE) gives the following annotation to this statement:

> Pricks grow within the skin shaped like millet or needles. Over time, they will turn black at the heads and can be as deep as one *fen*. (Except for the heads) they are yellowish white... This is popularly known as pricking powder (acne vulgaris).

When explaining the cause, *The Mirror* says, "This illness is produced by blood heat in the lung channel." However, there are also cases where the culprit is eating too much refined grain and foods with rich flavors. Fats and sweets generate dampness which transforms into heat. Damp heat may then become depressed internally, finding no way to drain out. It then surges up into the face, producing pricking powder or acne.

Treatment based on pattern discrimination

In terms of Chinese medicine there are three different patterns of acne:

1. Lung channel wind heat pattern: The face is flushed with red lesions which feel hot and painful. There may be pustules. The tongue is red with yellow fur, and the pulse is rapid and floating.

2. Stomach & intestine damp heat pattern: There are red lesions with nodular papules accompanied by constipation and short voidings of scanty, dark-colored urine. The tongue is red with yellow fur, and the pulse is rapid and slippery.

3. Liver depression & qi stagnation pattern: This is an obstinate, protracted pattern with dark purple lesions and vexation and agitation. It gets worse towards and at the end of the menstrual flow. The pulse is bowstring, and the tongue is dark in color with possible static spots or macules.

Treatment principles: Diffuse the lungs, drain heat and resolve toxins for lung channel wind heat. Clear and disinhibit dampness for stomach & intestine damp heat. Quicken the blood and dispel stasis for liver depression & qi stagnation. Select pertinent points on the yang channels as the ruling points.

Formula: *Shen Zhu* (GV 12) or *Fei Shu* (Bl 13) in case of lung heat. *Ling Tai* (GV 10) in case of stomach heat. *Ge Shu* (Bl 17) in case of liver stasis.

Treatment method: Needle using draining technique. Follow pricking by cupping to let out some blood.

Other choices:

1. Moxa the local pertinent points, the back transporting points, or the tip of the fist, *i.e.*, the metacarpophalangeal joint, of the middle finger 1 time each day.

2. Break the subcutaneous fiber(s) under the small spot(s) of abnormal color appearing on the upper back with a three-edged needle and then let out a bit of blood by pressing or cupping.

3. Prick with a three-edged needle or tap with a cutaneous needle *Da Zhui* (GV14) and then immediately perform cupping over it 2 times per week.

4. Perform puncturing, needle-implanting, or pressing at the auricular points Lung (MA-IC1), Kidney (MA), and Endocrine (MA-IC3). Add the points Spleen (MA) and Spirit Gate (MA-TF4) in case of copious seborrhea. Add Large Intestine (MA-SC4) in case of constipation. Add Liver (MA-SC5) and Subcortex (MA-AT1) in case of stagnant qi and blood stasis.

Case history: A male, aged 15, complained of cystic acne which had formed a sinus 10mm long with several cysts the size of an almond. His skin was oily. The patient had a predilection for fatty meat and had an impetuous character. The treatment principles were to clear heat and resolve toxins. The procedures included bleeding *Fei Shu* (Bl 13) and fire-needling the local lesions to help discharge accumulated secretion. One week later, the condition was under control. Continued treatment for a couple of months, 1 time per month, healed the sore completely without leaving a scar.

Reference: There is a report of 30 cases of acne treated by needling *Qu Chi* (LI 11). Twenty-nine were healed and one suspended treatment half way for an unidentifiable reason. The needling was performed with medium strong stimulation with 30 minutes of needle retention. Li Feng-bo: *Zhong Guo Zhen Jiu (Chin. Acu. & Mox.)* 1983; 4:39.

23
White Patch Wind (Vitiligo)

Treatment based on pattern discrimination

In terms of Chinese medicine, there are two different patterns:

1. Blood vacuity pattern: The white patch has no distinct boundaries and the patient suffers from weakness. There is a white facial complexion, a light red tongue body with thin, white fur, and a weak, fine pulse.

2. Blood stasis pattern: The white patch has distinct boundaries. The toungue is red with static spots or static macules on its sides, and the pulse is choppy.

Treatment principles: Boost the qi and quicken the blood

Formula: *Fei Shu* (Bl 13), *He Gu* (LI 4), *Qu Chi* (LI 11) and *San Yin Jiao* (Sp 6)

Treatment method: Puncture performing even supplementation and drainage with the needles retained for 30 minutes. Treat 1 time each day with 10 days equalling 1 course.

Explanation of the formula: Since the qi precedes and governs the blood, to treat blood diseases, one should focus on normalizing the qi. *Fei Shu* (Bl 13) connects directly with the lungs and thus is a point that can fulfil this task satisfactorily. *San Yin Jiao* (Sp 6) enriches the blood as well as transforms stasis. The color white is ascribed to lung metal. Therefore, it is necessary to boost the lungs. Because *He Gu* (LI 4) and *Qu Chi* (LI 11) are important points of the hand *yang ming* which has an exterior/interior relationship with the hand *tai yin* channel of the lungs, the lungs benefit from needling these two points.

Other choices:

1. Puncture or press the auricular points Endocrine (MA-IC3), Spirit Gate (MA-TF4), Lung (MA-IC1), Adrenal (MA), and Sympathesis (MA-AH7) 1 time each day.

2. Perform cutaneous needling at the locally affected part and/or the point White Patch Wind (*Bai Dian Feng*) which is located in the middle of the palmar crease of the second phalangeal joint of the middle finger.

3. Moxa the affected part 1 time each day with 15 treatments equalling 1 course.

References:

There is a report of a number of cases of vitiligo treated by means of moxaing with a mugwort roll over the affected part. All the cases studied were healed. In most cases, 28-36 treatments were required. Li Hong-fu: *Zhong Guo Zhen Jiu (Chin. Acu. & Mox.)* 1983; 3(3): 29.

There is another inspiring report from Sri Lanka. The patient studied was a female, aged 48, and was a teacher. Initially, she had a small white patch on her right thumb. She received treatment, but two years later, her vitiligo had spread over almost her entire body. This distressing condition had persisted for 12 years when she came to ask for a trial of acupuncture treatment. She looked depressed and listless, and she suffered from such troubles as insomnia and poor appetite. The treatment plan was designed on the basis of five phases theory. Since the skin was the victim and the skin is ascribed to metal, the points of the large intestine channel, *He Gu* (LI 4) and *Qu Chi* (LI 11) were selected as the ruling points. Metal is banked by earth. Therefore, an earth point, *i.e.*, a spleen channel point, was also chosen. It was *San Yin Jiao* (Sp 6). Metal restrains wood. If metal is exuberant, wood is affected. Based on this thinking, *Xing Jian* (Liv 2) was selected since it is a point on the liver channel. These points were electroacupunctured with gentle stimulation. In the first course consisting of 10 days, 1 treatment was given every day. In the second course, 1 treatment was given every other day. In the third course, 1 treatment was given every third day. From the fourth course on, 1 treatment was given every fifth day. By the end of the first course, the skin of the face had begun to change in color, and the patient experienced improvement in her sleep and appetite. As the courses went on, her skin color gradually was restored to normal from the upper to the lower part of the body. By the end of the fourth course, about 50% of the skin had been restored to its normal color. A.D.V. Premaratue: *(Am. J. Acupuncture)* 1980; Vol. 8 (3).

24
White Sore (Psoriasis)

In the old classics, this disease had quite a number of different names, for example, pine bark lichen, obstinate lichen, snake's flea, dry lichen, and white slough lichen. In Chinese medicine, *xian* or lichen is a general term for all species of pathological changes of the skin whose main characteristic is itching. In modern medicine, this disease is divided into four categories: psoriasis vulgaris, psoriasis pustulosus, psoriasis arthropathica, and erythrodermic psoriasis.

Disease causes, disease mechanisms

From the view point of Chinese medicine, psoriasis may be caused by blood heat and blood dryness. Blood heat and dryness may be a product of invading wind evils which become depressed within the body. Internally, it may result from depletion and detriment of the liver and kidneys, penetrating and controlling vessel loss of balance, or disharmony of the constructive and blood. Sometimes, however, it is impugned to an unhealthy diet, for example, eating too much acrid food.

Psoriasis is a persistent skin disease that recurs easily after being cured. However, acumoxatherapy has proven an effective treatment option for this disease.

Treatment based on pattern discrimination

Clinically, there are two patterns which should not be treated in the same way.

1. Wind dampness brewing heat pattern: At first, scattered red papules appear. Soon these papules coalesce into patches of various sizes and the skin becomes rough, shedding a small amount of thin scales. There is unbearable itching often accompanied by thirst, a dry mouth, vexation, restlessness, troubled sleep, a red tongue body with yellow fur, and a rapid, slippery or rapid, bowstring pulse.

Treatment principles: Dispel wind, clear heat, and disinhibit dampness

Formula: *Qu Chi* (LI 11), *Da Zhui* (GV 14), *Yin Ling Quan* (Sp 9) and *a shi* points

Treatment method: Needle the first three points using draining technique. Puncture 1-3 points in the center of the lesion and 3-10 points at the periphery, inserting the needles downward towards the center. Retain the needles for 30 minutes.

Explanation of the formula: *Qu Chi* (LI 11) and *Da Zhui* (GV 14) dispel wind and clear heat. *Yin Ling Quan* (Sp 9) is able to transform dampness. The local points are intended to free the network vessels and move the blood to stop itching.

2. Blood vacuity generating wind pattern: This is a very refractory, enduring pattern with skin thickening, roughening, and unbearable itching which gets worse at night. The tongue is pale with thin fur, and the pulse is fine.

Treatment principles: Nourish the blood, moisten dryness, and dispel wind

Formula: *He Gu* (LI 4), *Qu Chi* (LI 11), *Xue Hai* (Sp 10), *San Yin Jiao* (Sp 6), and *a shi* points

Treatment method: Needle the first four points using even manipulation, *i.e.*, non-draining/non-supplementing technique. The *a shi* points should be treated the same as instructed above.

Modifications: Add *Feng Shi* (GB 31) in case of severe itching. Add *Ge Shu* (Bl 17) and Hundred Worm Borrow (*Bai Chong Wo*), located 1 *cun* proximal to *Xue Hai* (Sp 10), in case of yin vacuity and blood dryness. Bleed the green-blue vein(s) behind the auricle of the ear in intractable cases.

Explanation of the formula: *Xue Hai* (Sp 10) and *San Yin Jiao* (Sp 6) can nourish the blood and moisten dryness. *Qu Chi* (LI 11) and *He Gu* (LI 4) dispel wind and stop itching.

Other choices:

1. Needle *Da Zhui* (GV 14), *Qu Chi* (LI 11), *San Li* (St 36), and *San Yin Jiao* (Sp 6) 1 time each day.

2. Prick *Fei Shu* (Bl 13) to let out a bit of blood by pressing after extracting the needle or, for a strong case, by means of cupping.

3. Prick every spinal joint from *Da Zhui* (GV 14) to *Yang Guan* (GV 3) with a three-edged needle, 2 times per week.

4. Puncture or press the auricular points Lung (MA-IC1), Endocrine (MA-IC3), and Spirit Gate (MA-TF4).

5. Perform cutaneous needling at *Fei Shu* (Bl 13) and the locally affected areas, 1 time every other day.

6. Moxa the local affected area over garlic.

Case history: A 14 year old male had psoriasis on his four limbs, his head, and his trunk with pustular acne on his face. The patient had received various treatments with no effect. The case was diagnosed as a lung heat pattern. The prescription included pricking and cupping *Fei Shu* (Bl 13) and administering a lung heat-clearing formula composed of Herba Seu Flos Schizonepetae Tenuifoliae (*Jing Jie*), Radix Ledebouriellae Divaricatae (*Fang Feng*), Radix Scutellariae Baicalensis (*Huang Qin*), Radix Angelicae Sinensis (*Dang Gui*), Rhizoma Coptidis Chinensis (*Huang Lian*), Radix Et Rhizoma Rhei (*Da Huang*), Periostracum Cicadae (*Chan Tui*), Fructus Gardeniae Jasminoidis (*Zhi Zi*), and uncooked Radix Rehmanniae (*Sheng Di*).

Note: Chinese acupuncturists typically combine Chinese medicinals with acumoxatherapy when treating psoriasis.

References:

There is a report of 240 cases of psoriasis treated by pricking the *Hua Tuo Jia Ji* or paravertebral points to let out a bit of blood. These points are located 5 *fen* bilateral to the spine. Two hundred twenty-two cases were healed, and 18 cases showed marked improvement. There were no recurrences on follow-up after one year. Zhang Lian-cheng: *Zhe Jiang Zhong Yi Za Zhi (Zhejiang Journal of C.M.)* 1990; 25(9):423.

In another report, 600 cases of psoriasis were treated by means of pricking followed by cupping at *Da Zhui* (GV 14), *Tao Dao* (GV 13), *Gan Shu* (Bl 18), and *Pi Shu* (Bl 20). The results were 401 successes; 115 cases showed marked improvement, and 84 were failures. Zhao Fu-yun: *Shan Xi Zhong Yi Za Zhi (Shanxi J. of C.M.)* 1982; (4):145.

25
Wet Foot Qi (Athelete's Foot)

This is usually a nasty yet mild malady. However, sometimes it can be very serious.

Disease causes, disease mechanisms

Downpouring damp heat is the evil qi in most cases. Either long exposure to a damp environment or dietary irregularity may be the cause of this damp heat. When damp heat lodges in the feet, it may steam the skin, causing itching and making the skin putrefy.

Treatment principles: Clear heat and disinhibit dampness in the early stages. Nourish blood and moisten dryness in the advanced stage.

Formula: *Yin Ling Quan* (Sp 9), *San Li* (St 36), and *Ba Feng* (M-LE-8)

Treatment method: Needle the first two points using draining technique. Then bleed the *Ba Feng* (M-LE-8) a bit.

Explanation of the formula: *Yin Ling Quan* (Sp 9) and *San Li* (St 36) in combination are able to clear heat from the blood and disinhibit dampness by fortifying the spleen and stomach, while the *Ba Feng* (M-LE-8) stops itching and courses the channels and network vessels to help eliminate damp heat evils.

Other choices:

1. Moxa the *Ba Feng* (M-LE-8) and the locally affected areas.

2. Fire-needling: This is often used in severe cases with infectious suppuration. First, one should strip the necrotic epidermis after dipping the foot in a solution of Cortex Phellodendri (*Huang Bai*) for 30 minutes. Next, moxa the local points. And finally, prick open the festering places with a red-hot needle to help discharge pus.

Case histories:

A male, aged 45, complained of infection in his left foot, the back of which was swollen with terrible ulceration between his toes. First, the white necrotic epidermis was stripped off after sterilization and dipping the foot in a solution of Cortex Phellodendri (*Huang Bai*). Then, fire-needling was applied to the necrotic places. The next day, his condition was a little better, but the swelling was still there. Moxibustion was performed at the local points, and *Qu Fu Sheng Ji San* (Dipel Rot & Generate Muscle [*i.e.*, Flesh] Powder) was applied to the infected parts. This powder is prepared from Gypsum Fibrosum (*Shi Gao*), Mercuric Oxide (*Hong Gong*), and Borneolum (*Bing Pian*). The case was healed after 20 days of treatment.

A male student, aged 22, complained of unbearable itching between the toes of his left foot which was swollen. The patient had been given antibiotics to no avail. Fire-needling was applied to discharge pus from the festering parts, and then bleeding was performed at the *Ba Feng* (M-LE-8). The next day, the swelling and itching had disappeared.

Reference: In a report of 100 cases of athlete's foot treated by electroacupuncturing *Yu Zhen* (Bl 11), the needle was retained for 30 minutes with strong stimulation. Forty-six cases were healed; 42 showed marked improvement; and 12 were failures. Song Jun-hui: *Zhong Guo Zhen Jiu (Chin. Acu. & Mox.)* 1985; 5(3): 16.

26
Wind Glossy Scalp (Alopecia Areata)

This condition is popularly known as ghost haircut since this disease may start all of a sudden, part of the head hair coming off overnight. However, alopecia areata may develop into total baldness (alopecia totalis) or general alopecia (alopecia universalis).

Disease causes, disease mechanisms

The Orthodox Gathering says:

> Wind glossy scalp is due to blood being too vacuous to follow qi to nourish the muscles and skin. Since the root of the hair is empty, patches of hair come off. The skin becomes shiny and itchy like worms crawling.

As a survey of 105 cases of alopecia the author has carried out shows, apparently emotional disturbance has something to do with over 70% of such cases. Such emotional factors include stress, worry, frustration, disappointment and depression, experience of fright, etc.

Treatment based on pattern discrimination

Past great medical figures have agreed that enriching and supplementing essence and blood should be given priority in the treatment of this disease. In modern times, Chinese practitioners prefer to use a combination of orally administered Chinese medicinals with acumoxatherapy and its variants, such as ear needling.

Theoretically wind gloss scalp is divided into four patterns:

1. Blood vacuity & exuberant wind pattern: This pattern is characterized by its sudden onset and slight itching accompanied by dizziness, insomnia, heart palpitations, and impaired memory. The tongue is pale with white fur, and the pulse is fine and rapid.

2. Liver-kidney insufficiency pattern: This pattern is characterized by its protracted course, no growth of new hair, and likely development of total or universal alopecia accompanied by dizziness, insomnia, ringing in the ears, aching and weakness of the low back and knees, impotence, seminal emission, and menstrual irregularity. The tongue is pale with little fur, and the pulse is fine and bowstring.

3. Qi stagnation & blood stasis pattern: This pattern can be protracted and is accompanied by headache, poor sleep, chest oppression, and a dull, somber facial complexion. The tongue is dark in color with static spots or macules and white fur. The pulse is fine and choppy.

4. Spleen vacuity with damp heat pattern: This pattern is characterized by a prickly itching on the head with copious oily secretion accompanied by diarrhea or loose stools and torpid intake. The tongue is slightly red, and the pulse is slippery.

However, as far as treatment with acumoxatherapy is concerned, the above four patterns are re-classified into only two patterns for practical purposes.

1. Yin vacuity & blood dryness pattern: This is distinguished by insomnia, irascibility, red tongue body with little fur, and a fine, rapid pulse.

Treatment principles: Enrich yin and moisten dryness; cool the blood and quiet the spirit

Formula: *Tai Xi* (Ki 3), *Xue Hai* (Sp 10), *Shen Men* (Ht 7), and local *a shi* points

Treatment method: Needle the first three points using supplementation through twirling. Perform encircling needling in the locally affected area.

Explanation of the formula: As the source point of the kidneys, *Tai Xi* (Ki 3) is particularly good at enriching yin and supplementing the kidneys and liver. *Xue Hai* (Sp 10) cools the blood and quiets the spirit. *Shen Men* (Ht 7), the source point of the heart channel, is able to supplement the heart and settle the orientation or emotions.

2. Wind heat pattern: Wind heat manifestations help identify this pattern. For example, the skin in the affected area is red and there is yellow tongue fur and a rapid, slippery pulse. There may also be dizziness.

Treatment principles: Course wind and dissipate heat

Formula: *Qu Chi* (LI 11), *Feng Chi* (GB 20), *He Gu* (LI 4), and local *a shi* points

Modifications: Add *Tai Xi* (Ki 3) and *Shen Shu* (Bl 23) in case of kidney vacuity. Add *San Li* (St 36) and *Tai Chong* (Liv 3) in case of blood vacuity. Add *Xing Jian* (Liv 2) and *Ge Shu* (Bl 17) in case of stagnant qi. Add *San Li* (St 36) and *Pi Shu* (Bl 20) in case of spleen vacuity.

Treatment method: Needle all the above using draining technique except for the *a shi* points which should be treated by the encircling method. Treat 1 time each day with 10 treatments equalling 1 course. As an alternative to rounding-up needling, one may insert two needles transversely from the periphery of the local lesion and make them cross one another in the center of the lesion, or one may insert four needles transversely from four corners of the lesion.

Other choices:

1. Tap with a cutaneous needle from *Ming Men* (GV 4) to *Da Zhui* (GV 14), the back transporting points of the five viscera, and the five channels on the head. Continue tapping until the skin turns red.

2. Moxa over ginger the points in the above formula and/or the local lesion.

3. Puncture or press the auricular points Kidney (MA), Lung (MA-IC1), Endocrine (MA-IC3), and Sympathetic (MA-AH7).

Note: Experience shows that psychotherapy is important to heal this disease completely. There are cases that heal by themselves without other treatment if psychotherapy is appropriate.

Case history: A male, aged 24, complained of alopecia on his head. Two months previously, hair on his head was found to come off in an area as large as a walnut, and the area gradually became larger. Now the entire head was bald. In addition, the patient suffered from low back pain, aversion to cold, insomnia, profuse dreaming, impotence, seminal emission, dizziness, and fatigue. His tongue was pale with white fur, and his pulse was weak in the cubit position. The diagnosis was alopecia totalis due to insufficiency of the liver and kidneys. The treatment procedures included tapping the bald area with a cutaneous needle along the routes of the five channels on the head and puncturing *Xin Shu* (Bl 15) and *Shen Shu* (Bl 23). One treatment was given every other day with 10 treatments equalling 1 course. After 2 months of such treatment, new black hair grew back.

Reference: The author has treated 105 cases of alopecia with needling in combination with psychotherapy. Fifty-six cases were healed; 32 showed marked improvement; and 17 were failures. The total effectiveness rate was 83.91%. The treatment procedures were tapping the affected areas with a cutaneous needle until the skin was red and puncturing pertinent points on the bladder channel and some other points according to individual signs and symptoms. For example, in case of severe itching, *Feng Chi* (GB 20) and *Feng Fu* (GV 16) were added. In case of insomina, a Quite Sleep (*An Mian*) point was added. (There are several of these and which one is not specified.) In case of kidney vacuity, *Shen Shu* (Bl 23) and *Tai Xi* (Ki 3) were added. If balding occured at the vertex, *Bai Hui* (GV 20) was added. If it occured in the temporal area, *Tou Wei* (St 8) was added. *Anthology of the '95 Italian International Acupuncture & Moxibustion Conference.*

Book Three: Animal Bites

1
Bee & Wasp Sting

Bee and wasp sting usually produces slight swelling and pain. However, sometimes it may result in serious generalized troubles, such as fever, aversion to cold, dizziness, and nausea. If the person stung is allergic to the bee toxins, anaphylactic shock or even death may result.

Treatment method: As to the treatment, the *Wai Ke Qi Xuan (Enlightening the Subtleties of External Medicine)* published in 1604 CE says:

> Bee sting carries toxins. The sting is embedded within the flesh; so (first) it should be pricked out. Then wash (the wound) with good wine to heal it.

In modern times, bee or wasp sting is usually treated by pricking the stung place with a three-edged needle to let out blood. To promote this bleeding, one may further perform cupping over the pricked point. In addition, tapping the affected part with a cutaneous needle is also effective. This tapping should continue until there is slight bleeding.

Case history: Once during field work, the author was accidentally stung by bees. There was redness and swelling in the places which were stung along with burning pain and prickly itching. Luckily, she had brought a cutaneous needle or (so-called) plum blossom needle with her. She tapped the painful and itchy places until they bled, and the stings were healed on the spot.

2
Poisonous Snake Bite

Thanatophidia (a type of poisonous snake) bite may be fatal as Chen Shi-duo said in his *Dong Tian Ao Zhi (The Occult Purport of Heaven [Observed] in the Cavern)* published in 1694 CE:

> Snake bite wound may be located on the foot, the head, the trunk, or the abdomen... In severe cases, the foot may be swollen as large as the head, the head may be swollen as large as a stone grinder, or the abdomen may be swollen as large as a winnow... When the toxic qi attacks the heart inwards, the wounded will die.

Treatment based on pattern discrimination

In Chinese medicine, the treatment plan is decided by the pattern. In the initial stage, when the toxins have not spread far and wide, there may be no serious generalized signs and symptoms. Shortly after, a wind fire pattern or a pattern of toxins attacking the heart may appear.

1. The initial stage

Treatment principles: Expel and resolve toxins

Treatment method: First of all, promptly tie a tourniquet around the part of the body proximal to the wound and perform careful debridement. Cut a cross with a knife or needle between the marks of the snake's fangs. Prick this cut to let out blood, and then needle the *Ba Feng* (M-LE-8) and *Ba Xie* (M-LE-22). To promote bleeding, one may perform cupping over the pricked points.

Reference: *The Orthodox Gathering* says:

> Within one day of a bite, one may soak the wound in hot urine and wash away the blood stasis (with this urine) from the (snake) tooth imprints. Then apply *Chan Su Bing* (Toad Cake) to the holes of the bite. Later, the wound will become a little pussy and then heal.

This cake is prepared from Camphora (*Zhang Nao*), Cinnabar (*Zhu Sha*), Venum Bufonis Bufonis (*Chan Su*), Reisna Olibani (*Ru Xiang*), Resina Myrrhae (*Mo Yao*), Realgar (*Xiong Huang*), Calomelas (*Qing Fen*), Semen Crotonis Tiglii (*Ba Dou*), and Secretio Moschi Moschiferi (*She Xiang*).

2. Wind fire pattern: In the wind fire pattern, there is local redness and swelling with pain accompanied by insensitivity, bleeding, or necrosis as well as such generalized signs and symptoms as dizziness, flowery or blurred vision, aversion to cold, fever, nausea, retching and vomiting, caligo, heart palpitations, shortness of breath, vexation and agitation, and a rapid, bowstring or rapid, surging pulse.

Treatment principles: Dispel wind and resolve toxins in case of predominant wind. Clear heat, cool the blood, and resolve toxins in case of predominant fire

Formulas: For the predominant wind type: *Feng Chi* (GB 20), *Feng Fu* (GV 16), *Shen Zhu* (GV 12), *Ling Tai* (GV 10), *Fei Shu* (Bl 13), *Yang Fu* (GB 38), *Yang Ling Quan* (GB 34), *Qu Chi* (LI 11), and *He Gu* (LI 4)

For the predominant fire type: *Da Zhui* (GV 14), *Shen Zhu* (GV 12), *Ling Tai* (GV 10), *Xue Hai* (Sp 10), *San Yin Jiao* (Sp 6), *Tai Xi* (Ki 3), *Ge Shu* (Bl 17), *Feng Fu* (GV 16)

Treatment method: Needle all the above using draining technique.

Explanation of the formulas: Wind toxins easily stir up liver wind. Therefore, it is urgently necessary to eliminate wind in the predominant wind type. *Feng Chi* (GB 20) and *Feng Fu* (GV 16) are used just to dispel wind, clear heat, and resolve toxins. In addition, these two points are able to arouse the brain and open the portals, brighten the eyes and boost the intelligence. The governing vessel is where the various yang channels meet. Therefore, draining it may drain fire heat toxins. For that reason, *Shen Zhu* (GV 12) and *Ling Tai* (GV 10) are selected to promote the flow of inhibited qi and blood and free the circulation of the channels. Because *Fei Shu* (Bl 13) is a point which has direct access to the lungs, it is able to best adjust the great qi or gathering qi. The gallbadder and liver channels have an exterior-interior relationship. Therefore, draining *Yang Fu* (GB 38) and *Yang Ling Quan* (GB 34) is intended to subdue liver wind, while *Qu Chi* (LI 11) and *He Gu* (LI 4) course and dissipate heat from the *yang ming*.

In the second type, *i.e.,* the predominant fire species, fire toxins have invaded the qi division and are beginning to attack the constructive and blood divisions. Therefore, treatment should first clear heat toxins from the blood. Based on this analysis, a yin channel should be the focus. Hence, the spleen channel points, *San Yin Jiao* (Sp 6) and *Xue Hai* (Sp 10), are chosen to clear fire heat from the three yin channels. Since *Ge Shu* (Bl 17) is an omnipotent point for any blood troubles, it is used to clear heat from the blood. When combined with *Tai Xi* (Ki 3), a point on the kidney water channel, its action of clearing fire is enhanced since *Tai Xi* is able to enrich water.

3. Toxins attacking the heart pattern: The pattern of toxins attacking the heart is characterized by high fever, clouded spirit, raving, agitation and restlessness, rapid, distressed, dyspneic breathing with rales, dry, black tongue fur, and a rapid, surging pulse.

Treatment principles: Clear heat and resolve toxins, sweep away phlegm and open the portals

Formula: *Nei Guan* (Per 6), *Shen Men* (Ht 7), *Ren Zhong* (GV 26), *Feng Long* (St 40), and *Xin Shu* (Bl 15)

Treatment method: Needle all the above points using draining technique.

Modifications: In the case of yang desertion manifesting as faint breathing, a cold body, and an expiring pulse, add *San Li* (St 36), *Guan Yuan* (CV 4), and *Qi Hai* (CV 6). Moxa the last two; needle and then moxa *San Li* (St 36).

Explanation of the formula: The first two points are used to rectify the heart channel and to quiet the heart spirit. They act synergistically when combined with *Ren Zhong* (GV 26) which is good at arousing the brain and opening the portals. *Feng Long* (St 40) is a point which has been proven effective for sweeping away phlegm and transforming turbidity. In Chinese medicine, conditions such as clouded spirit and raving are regarded as phlegm confounding the spirit or heart portals. *Guan Yuan* (CV 4) and *Qi Hai* (CV 6) are recognized as particularly capable points for rescuing yang and boosting the qi. Moxaing *San Li* (St 36) warms the center and rescues yang.

3
Rabid Dog Bite (Rabies)

Rabid dog bite is an important topic in many old medical classics where, for example, all the problems of incubation, first emergency aids, and other treatments are discussed. There is an interesting passage describing rabid dogs in *The Orthodox Gathering* which says:

> Rabies in dogs is a result of constant exposure to untimely abnormal (weather) qi when lying in the open day and night. When its heart is affected, its tongue will loll. When its liver is affected, its eyes become clouded. When its spleen is affected, it will drool from the mouth. When its lungs are affected, it is unable to bark. When its kidneys are affected, its tail will trail (along the ground). When its five viscera have (all) received the toxins, it becomes rabid. Because the rabid dog has been subject to yin and yang killing qi, it is capable of bringing injury to people.

Disease causes, disease mechanisms

Rabid dog bite carries extremely lethal toxins of wind evil and fire evil nature. Therefore, once these toxins find their way into the body, they progress with astounding swiftness. At first, they attack the muscles and channels, causing stagnation of the channels and vessels. Then the toxins attack the viscera and bowels, producing a series of severe pathologic changes in them. Soon afterwards, they attack the heart, driving the spirit into disorder and causing fear of wind and hydrophobia. As the toxins penetrate deeper, they engender wind at a fast speed. Stirring of liver wind then produces spasms and tremors. Finally, the qi of the five viscera expires and yin and yang separate from one another. Now death comes.

Treatment based on pattern discrimination

Rabid dog bite is divided into three main stages:

1. The initial stage: There is slight fever and headache, weakness, no appetite, aversion to wind and light, and constriction of the throat. The wound is itching, painful, and somewhat numb. There may be hypertonicity of the sinews. The tongue fur is white, and the pulse is floating.

Treatment principles: Resolve toxins through exterior effusion and lung diffusion, clear and drain the liver and gallbladder

Formula: *Da Zhui* (GV 14), *Feng Chi* (GB 20), *Qu Chi* (LI 11), *He Gu* (LI 4), *Fei Shu* (Bl 13), *Chi Ze* (Lu 5), *Yang Ling Quan* (GB 34), and *Tai Chong* (Liv 3)

Treatment method: Needle all the above points using draining technique and retain the needles for 20 minutes, strengthening stimulation at 5 minute intervals.

Explanation of the formula: The governing vessel is the sea of all the yang channels, while *Da Zhui* (GV 14) is the meeting point of all the yang channels. Therefore, draining this point resolves the exterior and clears heat toxins. In combination with it, *Feng Chi* (GB 20), *Qu Chi* (LI 11), and *He Gu* (LI 4) act synergistically in dissipating wind and resolving the exterior. *Fei Shu* (Bl 13) and *Qu Chi* (Lu 5) diffuse the lungs and disinhibit the throat. *Yang Ling Quan* (GB 34) is the meeting point of the sinews, while *Tai Chong* (Liv 3) is the source point of the liver channel which governs the sinews. These two points in combination clear and drain the liver and gallbladder to soothe the sinews.

Other choices:

1. Moxa the wound and then *Wai Qiu* (GB 36).

2. After debridement, prick the wound at a number of points and then perform cupping over them to let out blood.

2. The middle stage: The patient may run mad and suffer from vexation and agitation, restlessness, apprehensiveness, and/or aversion to the sight of water. Their voice is like barking or is hoarse. There is drooling from the mouth, copious spontaneous sweating, fever, thirst, and spasm and tremors arising on drinking. The tongue fur is slimy and yellow, and the pulse is rapid and bowstring, or rapid and surging.

Treatment principles: Quiet the spirit and calm the heart, arouse the brain and open the portals

Formula: *Da Zhui* (GV 14), *Bai Hui* (GV 20), *Ya Men* (GV 15), *Shui Gou* (GV 26), *Feng Fu* (GV 16), *Nei Guan* (Per 6), and *Feng Long* (St 40)

Treatment method: Needle all of the above points using draining technique.

Explanation of the formula: The governing vessel governs the yang of the whole body. Therefore, the points chosen on this vessel are capable of draining heat and settling mania. *Feng Fu* (GV 16) is particularly good at draining heat from the governing vessel and quieting the spirit. *Bai Hui* (GV 20) has direct access to the brain and hence is able to arouse it and open the portals.

Nei Guan (Per 6) is a point on the pericardium channel which is the guard of the heart. Therefore, it is able to drive heat evils from the pericardium and thus protect the heart. In combination with it, *Feng Long* (St 40) levels the stomach and downbears the turbidity that shuts the portals.

3. The advanced stage: In the advanced stage, spasms and tremors may stop, but there is generalized paralysis, upturned eyes, rapid, distressed, dyspneic breathing, and fecal and urinary block or incontinence. The pulse is very faint, expiring or near to expiring.

Treatment principles: Boost the qi, rescue yang, and secure yin

Formula: *Qi Hai* (CV 6), *Guan Yuan* (CV 4), *Qu Chi* (LI 11), *San Li* (St 36), *Feng Fu* (GV 16), *Feng Chi* (GB 20), *Lian Quan* (CV 23), and *Nei Guan* (Per 6)

Treatment method: Moxa *Qi Hai* (CV 6) and *Guan Yuan* (CV 4) over aconite cakes. Puncture *Feng Fu* (GV 16), inserting the needle obliquely downward towards the chin. Puncture *Feng Chi* (GB 20), inserting the needle towards the opposite side. When needling the above two points, one may extract (the needles) after having provoked strong stimulation. There is no need to retain the needles. Needle *San Li* (St 36) and *Qu Chi* (LI 11) using supplementing technique. It is better to make the needle sensation radiate to the tips of the toes and fingers. Needle *Nei Guan* (Per 6) and *Lian Quan* (CV 23) using draining technique.

Explanation of the formula: At this juncture, both the qi and blood are debilitated and the essence and spirit are exhausted even though there are still effulgent fire toxins. Therefore, it is urgently necessary to supplement and boost the righteous, while great efforts should be made to dispel toxins. *Qi Hai* (CV 6) and *Guan Yuan* (CV 4) are points able to boost the source qi and yang qi, and their action is enhanced when moxibustion is used. *San Li* (St 36) and *Qu Chi* (LI 11) are points on the *yang ming*. Needling them may free the *yang ming* channels to rescue yang and stem counterflow. *Feng Chi* (GB 20) and *Feng Fu* (GV 16) are points which have proven effective for suppressing wind and restoring qi expiry. When combined with *Lian Quan* (CV 23) and *Nei Guan* (Per 6), they can secure and restore the pulse and quiet the heart.

Case history: There is a modern report on the treatment of one case of rabies. The patient received an inoculation against rabies and then developed rabies. He suffered from insensitivity of the four limbs which gradually progressed into generalized paralysis. The treatment was composed of appropriate medication and needling. The points needled were *Qu Chi* (LI 11), *He Gu* (LI 4), *Shou San Li* (LI 10), *Zu San Li* (St 36), *Nei Guan* (Per 6), *Yang Ling Quan* (GB 34), *San Yin Jiao* (Sp 6), and *Tai Chong* (Liv 3). Needling was performed 4 times per week with 10-15 minutes of needle retention. Fifty-two treatments effected recovery. Yang Yuan-qing: *Shan Xi Zhong Yi Za Zhi (Shaanxi J. of C.M.)* 1982; (1):3.

Reference: From *The Simple Questions* on down, many medical classics have given various emergency treatments for rabid dog bite. A typical one contained in *The External Platform* is as follows: Once bitten by a rabid dog, one should immediately suck out the blood from the wound and then spit it out immediately. One should not in any case swallow down the blood. Then smash almonds and Folium Wendlandiae Uvariifoliae (*Shui Jin Shu*) and apply this mash to the wound. Moxa over the mash with 2 times 7, *i.e.*, 14, cones. From that day on, moxa it with 1-2 cones every day. Moxibustion over almond cakes should continue for 100 days.

Book Four: Orthopedics & Traumatology

1
Fracture

Disease causes, disease mechanisms

As far as the study of disease causes is concerned, there is a school founded by Zhang Zhong-jing holding that there are three kinds of disease causes. The most outstanding representative of this school was Chen Shi-ze (1131-1189 CE). In his work, the *San Yin Fang (Formulas Based on the Three Causes)*, he says:

> What is known as the six environmental excesses are cold, summerheat, dryness, dampness, wind, and heat, while what is spoken of as the seven affects are joy, anger, anxiety, thought, sorrow, fear, and fright... The neither internal nor external causes are hunger and overeating, shouting damaging the qi, straining the spirit to calculate and measure, tiring the sinews to the extreme... Incised wounds, sprains, fractures... are (also) neither internal nor external causes.

Therefore, it is clear that traumatology falls within the third kind of disease in terms of its cause. However, the three kinds of disease causes are often interrelated. In other words, in many cases, two or three different causes may underlie a condition.

Treatment based on pattern discrimination

Acupuncture and moxibustion cannot set a broken bone, but they may help with shock and swelling and to relieve pain, resolve spasm, strengthen the sinews, and facilitate the fixing of the broken bone in position. Acupuncture and moxibustion are usually performed after reduction of the fracture as an effective adjunct to facilitate rehabilitation. Roughly speaking, the treatment principles of fracture vary with the phases of the fracture:

1. The initial stage: In the initial stage, the focus of attention should be on quickening the blood and transforming stasis, dispersing swelling and relieving pain. In a word, priority is given to freeing the flow of the channels and network vessels. To free the channels and network vessels, one may needle local *a shi* points and points of the related channels. In addition to *a shi* and local points, the points often used for the above purposes are *He Gu* (LI 4), *Tai Chong* (Liv 3), *Xue Hai*

(Sp 10), and *Ge Shu* (Bl 17). If there is shock, it is urgently necessary to remedy this. To do this, one may arouse the brain and open the portals by needling *He Gu* (LI 4), *San Li* (St 36), and *Su Liao* (GV 25) or *Ren Zhong* (GV 26) and moxaing *Bai Hu*, (GV 20) and *Guan Yuan* (CV 4).

2. The middle stage: In the middle stage, when callus is being formed, one should focus the treatment on unblocking the channels and network vessels, transforming stasis and supplementing the liver and spleen. The points chosen for this purpose are *Pi Shu* (Bl 20), *Shen Shu* (Bl 23), *San Li* (St 36), *San Yin Jiao* (Sp 6), local *a shi* points, and pertinent points on the related channels.

3. The advanced stage: In the late stages, it is vital to strengthen the sinews and bones in order to promote fixing of the broken bone and to prevent dislocation or deformation. To do this, one may warm and further free the flow of the channels, replenish the liver, spleen, and kidneys, and supplement the qi and blood through needling local *a shi* points, *Guan Yuan* (CV 4), *San Yin Jiao* (Sp 6), *Yang Ling Quan* (GB 34), *San Li* (St 36), and pertinent points on the related channels.

In fracture, there is often binding in the channels which may further cause disharmony of the viscera and bowels. Hence, generalized troubles, such as constipation or diarrhea, menstrual irregularity, frequent voidings of urine, and seminal emission may appear.

The above is the treatment of fractures in general. However, because fractures may occur in different locations, one should adopt a flexible attitude in their treatment, selecting different teams of points in accordance with the particular location and nature of the fracture. The following is a detailed discussion of the treatment of fracture according to its location.

1. Fracture in the face

Formula: Local *a shi* points. Add *He Gu* (LI 4) and *Shou San Li* (LI 10) if the fracture occurs on the front of the head and face. Add *Wai Guan* (TB 5), *Feng Chi* (GB 20), and *Tai Chong* (Liv 3) if fracture occurs on the side of the face. Add *Lie Que* (Lu 7) and *Kun Lun* (Bl 60) if fracture occurs on the back of the head.

Modifications: Add *Si Shen Cong* (M-HN-1) and *Ren Zhong* (GV 26) to arouse the brain and open the portals and *San Li* (St 36) to boost the qi and blood in case of clouded spirit or loss of consciousness. Add *Ge Shu* (Bl 17) and *Qi Hai* (CV 6) in case of massive bleeding.

Treatment method: Moxa the wound and local *a shi* points; needle the others.

Explanation of the formula: There is a rhyme that says, "For troubles in the face, appeal to *He Gu* (LI 4), and to treat the back of the head *Lie Que* (Lu 7) never fails." Since the *yang ming* traverses the face, *He Gu* can cope with any disorders occuring in this part. *Lie Que* is a point on the lung channel. Although this channel does not go up to the head and face, *Lie Que* is a network point connecting the hand *tai yin* and hand *yang ming* channels. For that reason, it is also often among the options when treating diseases or wounds on the face and head.

When the side of the face is involved in fracture, the *shao yang* and *jue yin* channels are affected, and in most cases, there will be blood stasis which also involves the liver. This is because the liver stores the blood. Therefore, *Tai Chong* (Liv 3), selected by the method of points below to treat problems above, is expected to level the liver, harmonize the blood, and dispel blood stasis.

Case histories:

A male worker, aged 28, lost one of his eyes and had his nasal and orbital bones broken in an accident. After the fracture was reduced (literally, after the bones were straightened), the wounds became terribly swollen with copious secretion, and physiotherapy proved ineffective. My treatment was to moxa the local points. Moxaing 5 times succeeded in dispersing the swelling.

A male, aged 40, broke his temporal bone in a coal-mining accident. After the fracture was reduced, the patient suffered from fecal and urinary incontinence, hemiplegia, clouding of consciousness from time to time, unclear voice, irritability, a swollen face, deviated mouth and eyes, and red eyes. The treatment principles were to quicken the blood and transform stasis, free the flow of the channels and quicken the network vessels, arouse the brain and open the portals. The points needled were *Feng Chi* (GB 20), *Si Shen Cong* (M-HN-1), *Wai Guan* (TB 5), *Jue Gu* (GB 39), *Tai Chong* (Liv 3), *San Li* (St 36), and *Qu Chi* (LI 11). One week of treatment helped restore the patient's serenity. Two weeks later, the patient could rise up by himself. Two months of treatment enabled him to attend to daily life himself.

2. Skull fracture

Formula: *Feng Chi* (GB 20), *He Gu* (LI 4), *Tai Chong* (Liv 3), *Si Shen Cong* (M-HN-1), *Ren Zhong* (GV 26), and local *a shi* points

Modifications: Add *Zhi Yin* (Bl 67) in case of pain in the forehead. Add *Xia Xi* (GB 43) in case of one-sided headache. Add *Bai Hui* (GV 20) in case of pain in the vertex. Add *Tian Zhu* (Bl 10) and *Kun Lun* (Bl 60) in case of pain in the occipital region. Add *San Li* (St 36) and *Tai Chong* (Liv 3) in case of pain inside the head. Add *Lie Que* (Lu 7) in case of pain in the entire head. Add *Wai Guan* (TB 5) and *Yin Ling Quan* (Sp 9) in case of heavy headedness and headache.

Treatment method: In the initial stage, needle all the points. In the later stages, combine needling and moxibustion or merely use moxibustion.

Note: Since there may be conditions such as coma and bleeding from the seven portals—the nose, ears, mouth, and eyes—other points specific for these troubles should be chosen in addition.

3. Cervical fracture

Formula: In the initial stage: Needle *Feng Chi* (GB 20), *Wai Guan* (TB 5), and *Jue Gu* (GB 39). In the later stages: Needle and then moxa the *a shi* points, *Jue Gu* (GB 39), *Kun Lun* (Bl 60), and *Tai Xi* (Ki 3).

Explanation of the formula: The lateral side of the neck and back of the neck are ascribed to the *tai yang* and *shao yang* channels. *Feng Chi* (GB 20), therefore, is able to resolve hypertonicity and stop pain in this area. *Jue Gu* (GB 39) is the meeting point of the bone marrow. Therefore, it can achieve the feat of replenishing the essence and supplementing marrow to promote healing of the bone. As the source point of the kidney channel, *Tai Xi* (Ki 3) promotes the generation of new bone, strengthens the sinews, and invigorates the bone because the kidneys govern the bones. *Kun Lun* (Bl 60) is especially good at coursing and freeing the qi of the *tai yang* channel.

4. Sternum & rib fracture

Formula: *A shi* points, *He Gu* (LI 4), *Nei Guan* (Per 6), *Yang Ling Quan* (GB 34), *Ge Shu* (Bl 17), *Qu Chi* (LI 11), and *San Li* (St 36)

Treatment method: Needle these by turns, choosing 2-3 points each treatment, and treat 1 time each day.

Explanation of the formula: *Nei Guan* (Per 6) is a point which is specifically proven for troubles related to the chest. *He Gu* (LI 4) and *Qu Chi* (LI 11) are intended to supplement the lung qi or great qi to relieve pain. *Yang Ling Quan* (GB 34), a point on the gallbladder channel which runs across the chest, is effective in relieving chest and rib-side pain. *Ge Shu* (Bl 17), the meeting point of blood, is able to quicken the blood and transform stasis. *San Li* (St 36) and *Qu Chi* (LI 11), both sea points, are good at supplementing the qi and blood.

5. Thoracic & lumbar vertebra fracture & dislocation

Formula: In the initial stage: *Ren Zhong* (GV 26), *Hou Xi* (SI 3), *Su Liao* (GV 25), *Shen Shu* (Bl 23), *San Jiao Shu* (Bl 22), *Da Chang Shu* (Bl 25), *Zhong Ji* (CV 3), and *San Yin Jiao* (Sp 6). In the later stages: *Ji Zhong* (GV 6), *Zhi Yang* (GV 9), *Yao Shu* (GV 2), *Wei Zhong* (Bl 40), and the *Hua Tuo Jia Ji* points located 5 *fen* bilateral to the thoracic and lumbar spinous processes.

Treatment method: Needle using draining technique without retaining the needle 1 time each day during the initial stage, but 1 time every other day in the later stages. After that, also moxa the points.

Note: Experience proves that the combination of acupuncture and moxibustion with medication and massage therapy is necessary to achieve better results. The medicinal formula orally administered is composed of: Radix Angelicae Sinensis (*Dang Gui*), Radix Dipsaci (*Xu Duan*), Rhizoma Cibotii Barometsis (*Gou Ji*), Radix Astragali Membranacei (*Huang Qi*), Radix Lateralis Praeparatus Aconiti Carmichaeli (*Fu Zi*), Cortex Cinnamomi Cassiae (*Rou Gui*), Radix Cyathulae (*Chuan Niu Xi*), Ramus Loranthi Seu Visci (*Sang Ji Sheng*), and Rhizoma Drynariae (*Gu Sui Bu*).

Case history: A male, aged 40, sustained frontal, nasal, and spinal fractures in a traffic accident. After the patient had been hospitalized for 50 days, he requested acupuncture treatment because of refractory fecal and urinary incontinence, urethral infection, and constant spasm of his lower limbs and abdomen. In addition, the patient complained of cold in his external genitalia. The diagnosis was vacuity of both the spleen and kidneys. According to the principle that the branch should be treated first when it is urgent, the treatment of fecal and urinary incontinence was put above everything else. The method was to needle with supplementing technique and then moxa *Zhong Ji* (CV 3), *Shen Shu* (Bl 23), and *San Yin Jiao* (Sp 6). One treatment and his urination was under control, while the second treatment restored his control over defecation.

Then the focus of treatment turned to supplementing the kidneys and strengthening the bones, freeing the flow of the governing vessel and stopping pain, and harmonizing the qi and blood. The points needled were *Tai Xi* (Ki 3), *Shen Shu* (Bl 23), *Da Zhui* (GV 14), *Zhi Bian* (Bl 54), *Yao Shu* (GV 2), *Wei Zhong* (Bl 40), *Shou San Li* (LI 10), *Zu San Li* (St 36), *He Gu* (LI 4), *Tai Chong* (Liv 3), and *Bai Hui* (GV 20). The points moxaed were *Guan Yuan* (CV 4), *Ming Men* (GV 4), *Shen Shu* (Bl 23), and *Hui Yin* (CV 1). Besides the needling and moxibustion, massage therapy and oral medication were prescribed. The medicinal formula was *Jin Gui Shen Qi Wan* (*Golden Cabinet Kidney Qi Pills*). Treatment was given 1 time each day with 6 treatments equalling 1 course.

After 4 courses, his muscular strength improved noticeably, and the patient regained his ability to rise up and walk, with the help of others. The patient was discharged from the hospital but continued the combined treatment of acupuncture and moxibustion, medication, and massage therapy. At the end of 2 months treatment, his muscular strength had been restored basically to normal, and the patient could walk with an unsteady step by himself. The cold sensation in his perineum was considerably reduced. However, lower limbs spasms still persisted. Half a year later, all the remaining troubles had either substantially improved or disappeared. The patient is still under treatment.

6. Fracture of the extremities

Formula: Needle and moxa the local and adjacent points.

Case history: A 52 year old male broke his left fibula in a traffic accident. Two months after the fracture was reduced, the patient still suffered from inability to walk and swelling and pain in his left lower leg. The skin in the affected area was a somber green-blue color. X-rays revealed that there was still a seam at the point of resetting, but callus had already formed. The prescription was to needle and then moxa *Tiao Kou* (St 38), *San Li* (St 36), *Yin Ling Quan* (Sp 9), *Tai Xi* (Ki

3), and *Jue Gu* (GB 39) 1 time each day. By the end of 20 days of treatment, the swelling and pain were gone and the patient regained his ability to walk.

2
Wrenching of the Low Back (Acute Lumbar Sprain)

Disease causes, disease mechanisms

Concerning wrenching of the low back, in his *Jin Gui Yi (Supplement To [the Essentials from] the Golden Cabinet)*, the famous Chinese medical scholar, You Zai-jing (?-1749 CE), said:

> Low back pain due to blood stasis may be caused by wrenching and contusion when exerting oneself to lift weights. The low back is the key part in the body, and it is by its strength that (the body) flexes and extends and bends either forward or backward. Once it is hurt or injured, the blood vessels become stagnant and not freely flowing, while the channels and network vessels become congested and static. This then causes the person low back pain and inability to turn over. (Such low back pain is characterized) by a choppy pulse and excerbation at night.

Treatment principles: Free the flow of the channels and quicken the network vessels, move the qi and quicken the blood, dispel stasis and stop pain.

Treatment choices:

1. Puncture *Ren Zhong* (GV 26), in actuality inserting the needle horizontally at a point 1 *fen* to the left of *Ren Zhong*. Make sure that the tip of the needle comes out at the opposite side. Stimulate by withdrawing and thrusting forward the needle in this position.

2. Needle *Hou Xi* (SI 3) while the patient is asked to bend their low back forward and backward repeatedly. This is appropriate if injury is located on the route of the *tai yang* channel.

3. Needle *Yao Tong* (N-UE-19) while the patient is asked to bend their low back forward and backward repeatedly.

4. Needle *Shen Shu* (Bl 23) and *Ji Zhong* (GV 6).

5. Needle *Yang Lao* (SI 6) while the patient is asked to bend their low back forward and backward repeatedly. Then needle local *a shi* points while the patient lies on their stomach.

6. Prick the bulging green-blue vein at *Wei Zhong* (Bl 40) while the patient is standing.

7. Tap the painful place and the paravertebral points with a cutaneous needle until the skin is red.

Other choices:

Choose related points on the governing vessel and bladder channel as the ruling points.

References:

In one report on the treatment of low back wrenching with acupuncture, the method was to insert a 3-4 *cun* long needle at *Hou Xi* (SI 3) towards *He Gu* (LI 4), performing twirling drainage while the patient clenched their fist loosely. The needle was retained for 20-30 minutes or more in severe cases. While the needle was retained and rotated, the patient was asked to repeatedly squat down and rise up and to rotate the low back, particularly in the direction where movement was constrained. This needling was performed unilaterally on the same side as the affected part. If the pain was located right on the spine or bilaterally, *Hou Xi* was chosen bilaterally. Of 106 cases treated with this method, 103 were healed by 1-2 treatments. Two cases showed marked improvement, and 1 case had no response. The effectiveness rate was 98.98%. Liu Zhong-rong et al: *Zhong Guo Zhen Jiu (Chin. Acu. & Mox.)* 1995; (1):57.

There is another report on the treatment of 129 cases with acupuncture. The point chosen was *Shui Gou* (GV 26). While the needling was performed, the patient was instructed to move their low back about. The results were 114 successes. Fifteen other cases showed marked improvement. Zhang Yi-sheng: *Shan Dong Zhong Yi Za Zhi (Shandong J. of C.M.)* 1987; (4):51.

3
Forked Qi (Upper Back Sprain)

When wrenching happens to the lower back, it is called wrenching of the low back; when it occurs to the upper back, it is known as forked qi (*cha qi*). It modern terms, it amounts to thoracic vertebral facet disorder syndrome characterized by pain and aching in the chest, upper back, and rib-side region with a distended sensation or oppression. Forked qi is usually located on one side. In severe cases, there may be difficult breathing and constrained movement of the upper body.

Treatment choices:

1. Needle *Da Zhui* (GV 14) and the local *a shi*, i.e., tender points.

2. Needle *He Gu* (LI 4), *Fu Liu* (Ki 7), and *Kun Lun* (Bl 60).

4
Sinew Binding (Ganglion Cyst)

Disease causes, disease mechanisms

Sinew binding or nodulation is usually a product of gathered damp phlegm due to stagnant qi and blood. This stagnation of qi and blood is often ascribed to over taxation.

Treatment principles: Warm and free the flow of the qi and blood, quicken the network vessels and transform stasis. Choose the local *a shi* points as the ruling points.

Treatment choices:

1. Insert needles from the four corners at the edges of the nodulation towards the center of its base, using draining technique while the needles are retained or burning mugwort on the heads of the needles, *i.e.*, warm needle technique.

2. Insert a red-hot needle quickly into the center of the nodulation down to its base and then press out the fluid from the nodulation.

3. Moxa the center and boundary of the nodulation either directly or over ginger.

4. Massage therapy: Rub the nodulation until the skin is red. Then press it hard until it is dispersed. Bind up the dispersed nodulation lest it grow back again. And finally, fix the joint so that it is straight.

Case history: A female, aged 26 complained of a smooth, hard nodulation the size of a date in the middle of the back of her right wrist. A red-hot three-edged needle was inserted into the center of the nodulation. Then some sticky, semifluid substance was pressed out from the needle hole. Finally, the ganglion cyst was bound up tightly for 2 days. On follow-up after 2 years, there had been no relapse. The author has used this technique in 11 cases, of which only 1 had a relapse. All the rest healed completely.

Reference: There is a report on the treatment of 36 cases of ganglion cyst with fire-needling, of which 33 were healed and 3 had relapse. The needling was the same as in the case history above. Zhang Tong-liang: *Zhong Guo Zhen Jiu (Chin. Acu. & Mox.)* 1983; (3):3.

5
Heel Pain

Disease causes, disease mechanisms

Internally, heel pain is impugned to insufficiency of qi and blood and vacuity of the kidneys. The heels are liable to sustain insufficiency of the qi and blood because they are a remote part which is difficult for the qi and blood to access. Then why is this pain not ascribed to vacuity of some other viscus or viscera than the kidneys? Because the heels are within the reach of the foot *shao yin* channel. Heel pain of the internal pattern is usually accompanied and preceded by weak and aching knees, chilled limbs, diarrhea, impotence, a pale tongue, and a fine, deep pulse. Externally, cold and dampness may be responsible for this pain because they are yin in nature and hence likely to start from below. Thus the heel is a part of the body subject to them. In addition, knocks and falls may also cause heel pain.

Treatment based on pattern discrimination

In treating heel pain, one must identify different patterns by determining whether any other part of the foot than the heel is also involved. If, for example, the big toe is involved and the pain starts from there and ends in the heel, this is a yin pattern. Then one should choose *Zhong Du* (Liv 6), *Fu Liu* (Ki 7), and *Yin Ling Quan* (Sp 9). If the pain starts on the lateral side of the foot, one should choose *Yang Fu* (GB 38), *Jue Gu* (GB 39), *Yang Ling Quan* (GB 34), *Feng Shi* (GB 31), etc. If the pain is confined to the heel, then the following plan is appropriate.

Treatment principles: Supplement the kidneys and boost essence, free the flow of the channels and quicken the network vessels, nourish the blood and soften the sinews, scatter cold and eliminate dampness

Formula: *Tai Xi* (Ki 3), *Shui Quan* (Ki 5), *Pu Can* (Bl 61), *Kun Lun* (Bl 60), and local *a shi* point(s)

Treatment method: Use the point-joining method in needling *Tai Xi* (Great Ravine, KI 3) and *Kun Lun* (Bl 60), inserting the needle at *Tai Xi* towards *Kun Lun*. In puncturing the other points, insert the needles towards the center of the heel. It is equally good if these points are moxaed.

Explanation of the formula: To treat heel pain, it is vital to choose the pertinent points on the kidney channel and its associated yang channel, the foot *tai yang*. As their names suggest, *Tai Xi* (Ki 3) and *Shui Quan* (Water Spring, Ki 5) are points particularly good at supplementing water, which is as good as saying the kidneys. *Kun Lun* (Bl 60) is the river point of the foot *tai yang* channel and hence is able to free the flow of the channel qi of the kidneys especially when combined with the above two points on the kidney channel.

Other choices:

1. Moxa the following two groups of points alternately: A) *Ming Men* (GV 4), *Shen Shu* (Bl 23), and *Ci Liao* (Bl 32). B) *Guan Yuan* (CV 4), *Yin Gu* (Ki 10), and *Yong Quan* (Ki 1).

2. Needle *Cheng Shan* (Bl 57), *Cheng Jin* (Bl 56), *Xia Lian* (St 39), and *Kun Lun* (Bl 60).

3. Needle *Nei Ting* (St 44), *Pu Can* (Bl 61), and *Kun Lun* (Bl 60).

4. Press or puncture the auricular points Kidney (MA), Liver (MA-SC5), Heel (MA-AH1), Ankle (MA-AH2), and Spirit Gate (MA-TF1).

Case history: A female, aged 46, had had heel pain for half a year. When the patient came for acupuncture treatment, she was unable to walk because of the heel pain and also complained of low back pain. The case was diagnosed as a kidney vacuity pattern. The prescription was needling followed by moxibustion at *Shui Quan* (Ki 5), *Shen Shu* (Bl 23), and *Tai Xi* (Ki 3) joined to *Kun Lun* (Bl 60). In puncturing, the needles were retained for 20 minutes. Treatment was given 1 time each day. Seven treatments and the patient was healed.

References:

There is a report on the moxibustion treatment of heel pain. The procedures were to find tender points in the local area, dabbing on these a bit of medicinal wine for quickening the blood, and then moxaing these points with small cones of mugwort mixed with Borneol (*Bing Pian*), Realgar (*Xiong Huang*), and Secretio Moschi Moshciferi (*She Xiang*). When the patient felt very hot, the live cones were immediately put out in order to allow the hot qi to penetrate into the heel. This was done several times in 1 treatment. Fifty-six cases of heel pain were handled this way. Thirty-eight were healed; 14 showed marked improvement; and 4 got no effect. Yan Cui-lan: *Zhong Guo Zhong Yi Zheng Gu Shang Ke Za Zhi (Chinese J. of C. M. Orthopedics & Traumatology)* 1985; (5).

There is another report of the treatment of 15 cases by needling *Xia Guan* (St 7) bilaterally. After insertion, the needle caused a distended, numb sensation around the point, and while twirling manipulation was applied, the heel felt hot. Then the needle was retained for 30 minutes. Of the cases studied, 9 were healed, and 6 showed marked improvement. Ning Gai-rong: *Zhong Guo Zhen Jiu (Chin. Acu. & Mox.)* 1993; (5):36.

6
Tail Bone Pain

This trouble is scarcely seen in the medical classics. However, it is occasionally seen in clinical practice.

Disease causes, disease mechanisms

In most cases, this condition is caused by injury to the tail bone due to long sitting or trauma.

Treatment principles: Soothe the sinews and quicken the network vessels

Treatment method: Needle or perform flash moxibustion at *Chang Qiang* (GV 1) or the center of the painful area. In puncturing, the practitioner may perform lifting and thrusting drainage, retaining the needle for 10-15 minutes. The flash moxibustion technique is as follows: Light one end of a thin moxa roll. Put the burning end on the point for a brief moment. Then quickly put out the mugwort fire by pressing it against the point.

Case history: A male, aged 56, suffered a lot from pain in the tip of his tail bone after having travelled for a long time by train. The patient could not sit because of this pain. He was treated with the flash moxibustion method and the pain was relieved by 1 treatment.

Note: The author has treated more than 10 similar cases with the same method, all with success.

7
Damaged Sinews (Wrist & Ankle Sprain)

1. Wrist sprain

Disease causes, disease mechanisms

When speaking of wrist sprain, *The Origins* says:

> It is usually a sudden accidental damage. Because the qi and blood are subsequently blocked, they are no longer able to circulate and provide nourishment (to the sinews... To treat it,) one may perform massage therapy or qi conduction (*i.e., qi gong*) to restore the qi and blood.

Treatment principles: Dispel stasis and disperse swelling, soothe the sinews and stop pain

Formula: *Yang Chi* (TB 4), *Yang Xi* (LI 5), *Yang Gu* (SI 5), *He Gu* (LI 4), and local *a shi* point(s)

Treatment method: Needle these points using draining technique.

Explanation of the formula: *Yang Chi* (TB 4), *Yang Gu* (SI 5), and *Yang Xi* (LI 5) are each points on (one of) the three hand yang channels. As their names suggest, they are all points where the qi gathers and converges, and hence they are able to free the flow of the channels and quicken the network vessels. As *The Inner Classic* says, "Damaged qi manifests as pain and damaged form manifests as swelling." Either case requires, above all, freeing the flow of the qi.

Other choices:

1. Moxa the local *a shi* points. This, however, is effective only within 12 hours after the sprain.

2. Puncture or press the auricular points Wrist (MA-SF2), Adrenal (MA), and Spirit Gate (MA-TF1).

3. Electroacupuncture *Yang Xi* (LI 5) and *Yang Chi* (TB 4), retaining the needles for 20 minutes after obtaining the qi.

4. Massage therapy: First, rub the wrist with the palm or the palmar side of the fingers. Then rotate the wrist. And finally pinch *He Gu* (LI 4) and press *Wai Guan* (TB 5) and *Qu Ze* (Per 3). After these manipulations, apply a hot compress.

Note: Whenever I meet such a case, I use massage therapy as my first choice. This proves quite effective.

2. Ankle sprain

It is sprain of the lateral ligament which is commonly seen in clinical practice. This may manifest pain, swelling, and ecchymosis. If treated early enough, acupuncture and moxibustion are quite effective for relieving all of these symptoms.

Treatment principles: Soothe the sinews and quicken the network vessels, free the flow of the blood and transform stasis

Formula: *Shen Mai* (Bl 62), *Qiu Xu* (GB 40), *Shang Qiu* (Sp 5), *Jin Men* (Bl 63), *Zhao Hai* (Ki 6), *Zu San Li* (St 36), *Jie Xi* (St 41), *Yang Ling Quan* (GB 34), *Jue Gu* (GB 39), *Cheng Shan* (Bl 57), and local *a shi* point(s)

Treatment method: Needle without the need to perform supplementation or drainage. However, needle retention is required. Three days after the sprain, moxibustion can be used instead or in combination with needling.

Explanation of the formula: The combination of the local point *Jie Xi* (St 41) with the distant point *San Li* (St 36) is intended to free the *yang ming* completely. When the *yang ming* enjoys free circulation, it will provide sufficient qi and blood to repair the damaged sinews. The points on the gallbladder are selected to soften the sinews since the liver governs the sinews and the liver has an interior-exterior relationship with the gallbladder. Pertinent points of the foot *tai yang* should be included because, in most cases, the injured sinew runs within the reach of the qi of this channel.

Other choices:

1. Massage therapy: The procedures are as follows: First, rub the lateral aspect of the lower leg several times from the knee down to the ankle. Press *San Li* (St 36), *Yang Ling Quan* (GB 34), and *Jue Gu* (GB 39). Then pinch *Cheng Shan* (Bl 57). Gently rub the affected lateral side of the

ankle for several minutes. Rotate the ankle. Stretch the ankle with one hand holding the big toe and the other holding the heel. Finally, apply a hot compress as long as internal bleeding has stopped.

The above is appropriate in mild cases. If there is severe swelling around the ankle, one should only perform gentle rubbing of the leg, avoiding irritating the ankle. When the swelling has improved, one can do as instructed above. I always prefer this massage therapy as my first choice whenever I encounter a sprained ankle.

2. Perform cutaneous needling at the points prescribed for needling and moxaing above.

3. Apply externally *Da Huo Luo Dan* (Major Quicken the Network Vessels Elixir) or *Die Da Wan* (Fall & Knock Pills). Before applying these, one should make them into a semiliquid paste with water. These two pills are commercially available in the marketplace.

References:

There is a report on 31 cases of acute ankle sprain treated by puncturing *Yang Chi* (TB 4) alone on the affected side with 30 minutes of needle retention with satisfactory results. Mo Zhi-xiu: *Zhong Guo Zhen Jiu (Chin. Acu. & Mox.)* 1985; (6):8.

There is another report of 89 cases treated with needling the *Ba Feng* (M-LE-8) as the ruling points. In case of severe swelling, *San Li* (St 36) and *Chong Yang* (St 42) were added. It was desirable that the needle sensation reach the instep of the foot. All the cases so treated were healed. Chen Yuan-fa: *Zhong Guo Zhen Jiu (Chin. Acu. & Mox.)* 1987; (2):55.

8
Flaccid Body (Traumatic Paraplegia)

Disease causes, disease mechanisms

The Spiritual Pivot says:

> Following falls, the four limbs may become flaccid and flabby, unable to contract. This is called flaccid body.

The Simple Questions also devotes a passage to this trouble, which says, "After a person has a fall, malign blood may be retained internally, causing abdominal distention and fullness and inability to defecate or urinate." From the point of view of Chinese medicine, injury due to slips or falls very often involves the governing vessel. As a result, this vessel is plunged into disorder in terms of its qi and blood, and its network vessels become stagnant and blocked. Since the governing vessel is the sea of all the yang channels and is also connected with some other vessels, such as the penetrating and controlling vessels, once it is damaged, this or that vessel or yang channel will be affected. This then produces a variety of complex diseases. If a yang channel of the hand is involved, the upper limbs may be disabled and become insensitive. If the penetrating vessel is involved, atrophic muscles and inhibited joints may occur, for, as *The Simple Questions* says, "The penetrating vessel is the sea of the channels and vessels, governing percolation and irrigation of (all) the ravines and valleys." If the urinary bladder channel is involved, the bladder may dysfunction, causing urinary incontinence. If the large intestine channel is affected, problems with defecation will appear. If the disease persists long, the yin channels will also become involved, and the case will become even more complicated.

Treatment based on pattern discrimination

1. The early stage

Treatment principles: Course and free the flow of the channels and network vessels, quicken the blood and transform stasis

Formula: *Zhong Ji* (CV 3), *Gui Lai* (St 29), *Tian Shu* (St 25), *Ming Men* (GV 4), *Guan Yuan* (CV 4), and *Shen Shu* (Bl 23)

Treatment method: Needle the first four points. Needle and then moxa the last two.

2. The late stages

Treatment principles: Supplement the kidneys and invigorate yang, adjust the governing vessel and harmonize the qi and blood

Formula: *Da Zhui* (GV 14), *Ming Men* (GV 4), *Yao Shu* (GV 2), and *Guan Yuan* (CV 4)

Treatment method: Electroacupuncture all the above points except the last point which should be moxaed.

Modification of the above two formulas: Add *Bai Hui* (GV 20) and *Si Shen Cong* (M-HN-1) in case of mental complications. Add relevant points on the yang channels of the hand, particularly the hand *yang ming*, for example, *Shou San Li* (LI 10) and *He Gu* (LI 4), in case of dysfunction of the upper limbs. Add relevant points on the yang channels of the foot, particularly the foot *yang ming*, for example, *San Li* (St 36), *Bi Guan* (St 31), *Tai Chong* (Liv 3), *Jue Gu* (GB 39), and *Yang Ling Quan* (GB 34), in case of dysfunction of the lower limbs. Moxa *Shen Shu* (Bl 23) in case of fecal and urinary troubles.

Explanation of the above two formulas: *Da Zhui* (GV 14), *Ming Men* (GV 4), and *Yao Shu* (GV 2) are points on the governing vessel which is able to bear up the yang qi and hence to quicken the viscera and bowels. *Zhong Ji* (CV 3) is the alarm point of the urinary bladder, while *Shen Shu* (Bl 23) is the back transporting point of the kidneys which are in control of defecation and urination. The combination of these two points may unblock defecation and urination. *Tian Shu* (St 25) is the alarm point of the large intestine and, therefore, is able to restore the conveyance of the bowels and free the flow of the abdominal qi. *Bai Hui* (GV 20) is able to elevate the yang qi, while *Si Shen Cong* (M-HN-1) arouses the brain and opens the portals. The points of the hand and foot *yang ming* are proven points for wilting or paraplegia. As *The Spiritual Pivot* says, "To treat wilting, one should choose solely the *yang ming*." These points are able not only to supplement and boost the qi and blood but to quicken the channels and network vessels. *Yang Ling Quan* (GB 34) is the meeting point of the sinews, while *Jue Gu* (GB 39) is the meeting point of the bone marrow. Since this disease is due to damage of the governing vessel involving the yang channels, the yang qi must have stopped ascending. This results in withered sinews and bones. Therefore, these two points are apparently necessary. *Tai Chong* (Liv 3) is the source point of the liver and kidney qi and is also a meeting point with the penetrating vessel. To replenish the qi and blood, this point is chosen to supplement the penetrating vessel, the sea of all the channels, and the liver which governs the blood and the sinews. All the above points form a team which is particularly good at rectifying the blood and boosting the essence as a root treatment.

Flaccid Body (Traumatic Paraplegia)

Other choices:

1. Perform cutaneous needling paravertebrally and along the route of the pertinent channels on the limbs.

2. Moxa *Guan Yuan* (CV 4), *Shen Shu* (Bl 23), *Ming Men* (GV 4), *Pi Shu* (Bl 20), and *Zhang Men* (Liv 13).

Explanation of the formula: *Pi Shu* (Bl 20) is a point where the *tai yin* channel qi pours in, and *Zhang Men* (Liv 13) is the alarm point of the spleen. The combination of the back transporting and ventral alarm points of the spleen is able to supplement the central qi which is the supplier of qi and essence for all of the viscera and bowels. *Shen Shu* (Bl 23), *Guan Yuan* (CV 4), and *Ming Men* (GV 4) are intended to secure the source of generation and transformation. When the former and latter heaven or prenatal and postnatal qi are both supplemented and boosted, the root of life is protected. In sum, this team of points is a means of banking up the source and fortifying the root to treat the disease.

Case history: A male, aged 40, was a case of high quadriplegia. The patient had been involved in a traffic accident and, after emergency treatment, had become paralyzed of his four limbs. When he came for acupuncture treatment, he suffered a lot from incessant spasms of his limb muscles and abdominal straight muscles and severe urinary and fecal blockage. This could only be relieved by purgatives and catheterization which had produced suppurative infection in the urethra.

A treatment plan was immediately decided upon to first handle the branches, that is, the fecal and urinary blockage. The catheter and purgatives were abandoned. Needling was performed at *Zhong Ji* (CV 3), *Guan Yuan* (CV 4), *Shen Shu* (Bl 23), *Ming Men* (GV 4), *Tian Shu* (St 25), *San Li* (St 36), *Tai Chong* (Liv 3), *Yang Ling Quan* (GB 34), and *Jue Gu* (GB 39). The first four points were moxaed following the needling. Treatment was given daily. After the first treatment, the patient voided urine without any aid for the first time in the past scores of days. Three treatments enabled him to evacuate stools by himself. After 7 sessions, his urination and defecation were restored to normal. With it, the motor function of his four limbs improved a little. Then the following group of points were used: *Da Zhui* (GV 14), *Ming Men* (GV 4), *Yao Shu* (GV 2), *Zhi Bian* (Bl 54), *Wei Zhong* (Bl 40), *Jian Yu* (LI 15), *Shou San Li* (LI 10), *Wai Guan* (TB 5), *He Gu* (LI 4), *San Li* (St 36), *Jue Gu* (GB 39), *Tai Chong* (Liv 3), *Tian Shu* (St 25), and *Guan Yuan* (CV 4). After 1 month of treatment, the patient could turn over in bed and sit up. The same treatment continued, combined with massage therapy and oral administration of formulas of medicinals to supplement the kidneys and liver and strengthen the sinews and the bones. Three months after, the patient could walk 3 kilometers without any help. At present, the patient is still under treatment because some disorders remain to be cured, including impotence, occasional spasms of the lower limbs, and minor dysfunction of the hands.

Note: In the author's experience, some cases of traumatic paraplegia may be highly amenable to acumoxatherapy, especially if the treatment is carried out early enough. However, other cases seem recalcitrant, particularly those that have sustained substantial or organic lesions of the spinal marrow.

Book Five: Impediment

In Chinese, the word impediment means block. *The Spiritual Pivot* says, "The disease (of block) is named wind if it is located in the yang but impediment if it is located in the yin." Impediment in fact is a multivalent term. In *The Inner Classic*, there are a great number of passages devoted to the discussion of impediment. In sum, this term may refer to:

1. Stagnation or constriction, for instance, food impediment, a syndrome centering around the liver qi offending the stomach with food failing to descend, and throat impediment, whose main signs are sore throat and hoarse voice due to congestion of the throat.

2. Insensitivity of the skin and the flesh, for example, obstinate impediment, which may be caused by accumulated wind dampness forming blockage to the channels and network vessels in the defensive division.

3. Any condition of pain due to blocked qi and blood, like arthritis.

The viscera may also fall victim to impediment, and hence there is heart impediment, liver impediment, lung impediment, etc. which lie outside the scope of this work. Externally, impediment is divided into five categories by the depth it affects, namely, the skin, the sinews, the flesh, the bones, and the vessels. When viewed in terms of its characteristic clinical signs and symptoms, it may be differentiated as migratory, multiple, fixed, etc. And in relation to its location, we may have chest impediment, shoulder impediment, elbow impediment, etc.

The discussion herein is limited to that species of impediment which manifests as pain in the muscles, sinews, or joints, possibly accompanied by numbness, heaviness, and swelling due to inhibited qi and blood caused in turn by invasion of external evils or phlegm rheum collecting and gathering.

Disease causes, disease mechanisms

As in many other kinds of disease, it is righteous qi vacuity that provides a chance for external evils to invade and thus cause impediment. These invading evils are wind, cold, and dampness. If wind is the predominant factor, then impediment will take after wind and be constantly on the move. This species is also called migratory impediment. If cold is the predominant factor, then the qi and blood are congealed and the vessels contract, producing much pain. Therefore, this species is called painful impediment. If dampness is the predominant factor, then because dampness is sluggish, this species of impediment is characterized by fixed pain and heaviness of the muscles. Hence it is called fixed impediment. Cold and dampness, when depressed, may transform into heat, and hence cause heat pattern impediment.

1
Exposed Shoulder Wind (Periarthritis of the Shoulder)

Disease causes, disease mechanisms

As its name suggests, this disease is caused by exposure of the shoulder to wind cold which congeals and impedes the circulation of the qi and blood, forming block.

Treatment based on pattern discrimination

In exposed shoulder wind, the muscles are damaged. In the initial stage, there is chilling and pain in the shoulder which may involve the upper arm, neck, and even the fingers. In a later stage, the affected muscles become rigid and thinner, while cold and pain still remain. In the advanced stage, the pain and chilling may get better, but the affected joint becomes rigid and the muscles atrophic.

In Chinese medicine, exposed shoulder wind is classified in accordance with the channels. If the anterior area of the shoulder, for example, the area around *Zhong Fu* (Lu 1) is affected most conspicuously, this is a *tai yin* pattern. If the lateral side, for example, the area around *Jian Yu* (LI 15) is affected most conspicuously, this is a *yang ming* pattern. If the posterior area is affected most conspicuously, this is a *tai yang* pattern.

In most cases, wind is the predominant factor causing this disease. If the shoulder pain is deep in the bone and relievable by heat, then the main culprit is cold. Dampness is an evil that is most likely to damage the flesh. Therefore, if it is the prevailing evil, then the shoulder pain is found fixed in a certain area, mainly in the muscles and flesh, and there is possibly swelling.

Treatment principles: Warm the channels and scatter cold, dispel wind and eliminate dampness, strengthen the sinews and bones. Select relevant points on the three yang channels of the hand as the ruling points.

Formula: *Jian Yu* (LI 15), *Jian Zhen* (SI 9), *Bi Nao* (LI 14), *Qu Chi* (LI 11), *He Gu* (LI 4), and *Tiao Kou* (St 38)

Modifications: Add *Feng Chi* (GB 20) and *Wai Guan* (TB 5) in case of prevailing wind. Add *Jian Liao* (TB 14) and *Nao Shu* (SI 10) using warm needling in case of prevailing cold. Add *Yin Ling Quan* (Sp 9) and *San Li* (St 36) in case of prevailing dampness. Add *Chi Ze* (Lu 5) and *Yin Ling Quan* (Sp 9) for the *tai yin* pattern. Add *San Li* (St 36) and *Yang Ling Quan* (GB 34) for the *yang ming* and *shao yang* patterns. Add *Hou Xi* (SI 3) and *Tiao Kou* (St 38), inserting the needles towards *Cheng Shan* (Bl 57) for the *tai yang* pattern.

Treatment method: Except as otherwise instructed above, needle all these points using draining technique. Moxibustion may be performed in addition to or instead of needling.

Other choices:

1. Point-joining: Insert the needle at *Tiao Kou* (St 38) towards *Cheng Shan* (Bl 57), and *Yang Ling Quan* (GB 34) towards *Yin Ling Quan* (Sp 9). Ask the patient to move the affected shoulder while the needles are retained.

2. Puncture or press the auricular points Shoulder (MA-SF4), Clavicle (MA-SF5), Adrenal (MA), and the tender auricular point(s).

3. Moxa *Jian Yu* (LI 15), *Jian Liao* (TB 14), and local *a shi* points.

4. Electroacupuncture the points prescribed for moxaing immediately above.

5. Perform pricking, cupping, or cutaneous needling at the local tender point(s).

6. Massage therapy: The focuses are around *Jian Yu* (LI 15), *Jian Zhen* (SI 9), *Jian Zhong Shu* (SI 15), *Bing Feng* (SI 12), and *Tian Zong* (SI 11). The techniques include rubbing, pressing, pinching, pulling, rocking, scrubbing, and kneading.

Case history: A female, aged 51, complained of pain in the anterior part of her right shoulder which was exacerbated when the arm stretched backwards or in cold weather. Medications of different types had proven to have little effect. This was diagnosed as a cold pattern of the *yang ming* channel. *Jian Yu* (LI 15), *Bi Nao* (LI 14), and *Qu Chi* (LI 11) were punctured with mugwort being burnt on the heads of the needles while they were being retained. Additionally, after extraction of the needles, cupping was performed over the points needled. Treatment was given 1 time each day, and 10 treatments relieved the pain altogether.

References:

There is a report on treatment of 70 cases of exposed shoulder wind with combined needling and cupping. The treatment procedures were as follows: With the patient in a sitting position, the practitioner located and punctured the 2-3 most tender points to a depth of 2-3 *cun* with the needles retained for 20 minutes. After extraction, cupping was performed at the needled points to better provoke bleeding. Treatment was given 1 time each day, with 10 treatments equalling 1 course. By the end of the first course, the pain was much relieved in all the cases, and, by the end of the second course, none of the cases was left unhealed. Chen Ming *et al: Zhong Guo Zhen Jiu (Chin. Acu. & Mox.)* 1996; (2):14.

There is another report of fire-needling treatment of exposed shoulder wind. First of all, the practitioner chose 3-6 tender points and then thrust a red-hot needle quickly into the points one by one. The needle was not retained. Two such treatments achieved marked improvement in all 50 cases, of which 40 were healed completely. Meng Guo-chen: *Zhong Guo Zhen Jiu (Chin. Acu. & Mox.)* 1996; (1):26.

2
Taxed Elbow (Tennis Elbow)

Disease causes, disease mechanisms

This disorder is due to taxation detriment of the elbow with wind cold often conspiring in working up the trouble. It usually progresses slowly and easily recurs even after it is healed.

Treatment principles: Soothe the sinews and quicken the network vessels, nourish the blood and dispel stasis. The point selection principle is to combine the local points with distant points on the hand *yang ming* channel and/or a related channel.

Formula: *Zhou Liao* (LI 12), *Shou San Li* (LI 10), *Shou Wu Li* (LI 13), *He Gu* (LI 4), and local *a shi* points

Treatment method: Needle them all using draining technique.

Other choices:

1. Needle the point 1 *cun* proximal to *Yang Ling Quan* (GB 34) on the healthy side and ask the patient to move the elbow while the needle is retained.

2. Prick the tender points at the affected elbow to let out a bit of blood 1 time every other day, or needle and then moxa the tender points.

Reference: There is a report on the treatment of 50 cases of taxed elbow with moxibustion. The practitioner first found the tender points at the affected elbow, and, after dabbing some garlic juice on them, moxaed them each with three mugwort cones. The patient was asked to avoid straining the elbow for days to come. The results were 32 successes; 16 cases showed marked improvement; but 2 had no effect. The total effectiveness rate was 96%. Chen Li-qu: *Zhong Guo Zhen Jiu (Chin. Acu. & Mox.)* 1996; (3):26.

3
Jumping Round Wind (Sciatica)

This disease also falls within the category of impediment, having many different names in the old classics, such as lumbar leg pain, foot wilting, thigh wind, and thigh forked wind.

Disease causes, disease mechanisms

Jumping round wind is produced by wind cold which, after invading the hip and leg, transforms into heat, causing pain.

Treatment based on pattern discrimination

As in the case of exposed shoulder wind, jumping round wind is classified into several patterns in accordance with the affected channels. If, for example, the pain radiates from the hip joint down the anterio-lateral aspect of the leg, this is a *yang ming* pattern since that is the route of the foot *yang ming* channel. If the pain extends along the posterio-lateral aspect of the leg, then this is a *shao yang* pattern. The other patterns can be inferred in the same way.

Treatment principles: Warm the channels and free the flow of the network vessels, dispel wind and scatter cold. Treat the pertinent points on the related channel.

Formula: For the *tai yang* pattern: *Zhi Bian* (Bl 54), *Da Chang Shu* (Bl 25), *Cheng Fu* (Bl 36), *Wei Zhong* (Bl 40), *Cheng Shan* (Bl 57), and *Kun Lun* (Bl 60). For the *shao yang* pattern: *Huan Tiao* (GB 30), *Yang Ling Quan* (GB 34), *Feng Shi* (GB 31), and *Xuan Zhong* (GB 39). For the *yang ming* pattern: *Bi Guan* (St 31), *Fu Tu* (St 32), *San Li* (St 36), and *Feng Long* (St 40).

Treatment method: Needle using draining technique. The needle sensation should be extended to the toes. For a pattern of prevailing cold, it is better to needle and then moxa or to simply moxa. Electroacupuncture may be used instead.

Other choices:

1. Moxa directly or over ginger the local *a shi* points, the *Ba Liao* (Bl 31-34), *Zhi Bian* (Bl 54), *Shen Shu* (Bl 23), *Yao Yang Guan* (GV 3), and *Huan Tiao* (GB 30). These points may be needled and then moxaed in a single treatment.

2. Prick the local tender points and the minute vessels at *Shang Liao* (Bl 31), *Wei Zhong* (Bl 40), and *Wei Yang* (Bl 39). Then cup to let out a bit of blood.

Case history: A male, aged 46, was diagnosed with sciatica. He complained of pain in his left hip and leg which was refactory to pain-killers. I applied electroacupuncture, and 1 treatment relieved the pain considerably. One week of treatment effected a complete recovery.

Note: The author's clinical experience shows that electroacupuncture is a good alternative for sciatica and is particularly good for sciatic stem neuralgia. It offers but little help for sciatic root neuralgia or sciatica due to herniated disk. The author often chooses *Huan Tiao* (GB 30) and *Yang Ling Quan* (GB 34) for the *shao yang* pattern, and *Zhi Bian* (Bl 54) and *Cheng Shan* (Bl 57) for the *tai yang* pattern.

Reference: There is a report of the warm needling treatment of 200 cases of sciatica. The points prescribed were *Da Chang Shu* (Bl 25), *Guan Yuan Shu* (Bl 26), *Zhi Bian* (Bl 54), *Yin Men* (Bl 37), *Wei Zhong* (Bl 40), *Cheng Shan* (Bl 57), *Kun Lun* (Bl 60), *Huan Tiao* (GB 30), *Yang Ling Quan* (GB 34), *Xuan Zhong* (GB 39), and *Qiu Xu* (GB 40). While the needles were in position, a section of mugwort stalk was fixed to and burned on the head of each of the needles. This method resulted in the complete recovery of 152 cases, brought marked effect to 28 cases, and yielded improvement in 12 cases. Eight cases reported no effect. The total effectiveness rate was 96%. Xu Da-ren: *Zhong Guo Zhen Jiu (Chin. Acu. & Mox.)* 1993; (5):15.

4
Skin Impediment (Cutaneous Neuritis) (1)

In the old medical classics, skin impediment also appears under the name of fixed impediment (*zhuo bi*). It most often occurs in the lateral aspect of the thigh. It is characterized by numbness or a worm-wriggling sensation in the skin, possibly with aching.

Disease causes, disease mechanisms

If the righteous qi is vacuous so as to leave the interstices vacant and open, wind together with cold and/or dampness may take the advantage to invade the foot *shao yang* and *yang ming* in the thigh. This causes blockage or stagnation of the qi and blood there. There are cases, however, where stagnation of the qi and blood is caused by falls or knocks, *i.e.*, traumatic injury.

Treatment principles: Warm the channels and free the flow of the network vessels, quicken the blood and transform stasis, dispel wind, scatter cold, and eliminate dampness as necessary. Select pertinent points on the foot *yang ming* and *shao yang* channels as the ruling points.

Formula: *Feng Shi* (GB 31), *Bi Guan* (St 31), *Fu Tu* (St 32), *Liang Qiu* (St 34), *Yin Shi* (St 33), *Xue Hai* (Sp 10), and local *a shi* points

Treatment method: Needle *Feng Shi* (GB 31), *Yin Shi* (St 33), and *Xue Hai* (Sp 10) using lifting and thrusting drainage. Needle *Bi Guan* (St 31), *Fu Tu* (St 32), and *Liang Qiu* (St 34) using twirling drainage. Tap the *a shi* points with a cutaneous needle until there is bleeding or moxa them.

Explanation of the formula: *Feng Shi* (GB 31) is a point on the foot *shao yang*. It is miraculous for driving wind out from the thigh. The selection of *Xue Hai* (Sp 10) is based on the principle that, "The blood should be treated first when wind is to be treated" and that once the blood is moved, wind will die down by itself. *Bi Guan* (St 31) and the other points on the *yang ming* are important because, in order to free the qi and blood, especially in the thigh, one has to use the foot *yang ming* which is abundant in both qi and blood.

Other choices:

1. Perform cutaneous needling 1 time each day on the affected area until the skin becomes red or there is slight bleeding.

2. Perform sliding cupping. After dabbing some oil on the affected area, start cupping, sliding the cup up and down without letting any air in.

3. Needle *Feng Shi* (GB 31) and *Yin Shi* (St 33) or *He Gu* (LI 4) and *Tai Yuan* (Lu 9).

Case history: A male, aged 45, complained of numbness and a sensation of ants crawling on the skin of the anterio-lateral aspect of his thigh. The treatment prescribed was cutaneous needling followed by cupping. Five treatments brought relief.

References:

There is a report on the treatment of 85 cases of lateral femoral cutaneous neuritis with water point-injection. One tenth to 0.5ml of water was injected at the numbest point(s) or the upper and lower ends of the numb area 1 time every other day. Three treatments equalled 1 course. After 1-2 courses, all the cases were healed. On follow-up after 1 year, not a single case had relapsed. Liu Wen-ying: *Si Chuan Zhong Yi (Sichuan Chinese.Medicine)* 1985; (3):11. (*Bi Guan* (St 31) and *Feng Shi* (GB 31) may also be chosen for water injection.)

There is another report of 40 cases of lateral femoral cutaneous neuritis treated by means of vessel-pricking and cupping. The treatment steps were to tap with a plum blossom needle along the line from *Bi Guan* (St 31) to *Liang Qiu* (St 34) and from *Feng Chi* (GB 31) to *Xi Yang Guan* (GB 33) until the skin became red or there was slight bleeding. Then cupping was preformed in the same places using large cups to further produce bleeding. The total amount of the blood let out was 3-5ml. After 10 treatments, 30 of the cases studied had recovered; 5 showed effect; and 1 had no response. The effectiveness rate was 98%. Zhang Xiao-ping: *Shang Hai Zhen Jiu Za Zhi (Shanghai J. of Acu. & Mox.)* 1994; 13 (6):268.

5
Skin Impediment (Localized & Systemic Scleroderma) (2)

This is a disease of fibrosis and sclerosis of the dermal tissues which may eventually develop into atrophy and is accompanied by pain in the affected joints. In severe, enduring cases, it may advance further so as to involve the internal viscera and bowels, resulting in, for example, intestinal impediment or bladder impediment.

Disease causes, disease mechanisms

Originally, this disease is due to insufficient kidney yang or yang vacuity of the spleen and stomach. Subsequently, the defensive becomes weak and the interstices loose, and vacuity of the qi and blood arises. On the one hand, wind, cold, and damp evils take the advantage of this vacuity to invade, and, on the other, the qi and blood are sluggish and unable to provide sufficient supplies of nourishments to the skin and muscles. Therefore, the skin and muscles become hard, dry, and numb.

Treatment based on pattern discrimination

In modern medicine, this disease is divided into two categories, localized and systemic scleroderma, while in Chinese medicine, it is identified as six patterns.

1. Wind dampness pattern: This pattern, which is mainly due to invading wind dampness, is largely an external pattern. It is characterized by a waxy, bright complexion of the affected skin with no noticeable pain or itching. The pulse is floating and slippery.

Treatment principles: Dispel wind and eliminate dampness, free the flow of the network vessels and harmonize the blood

Formula: *Qu Chi* (LI 11), *He Gu* (LI 4), *Xue Hai* (Sp 10), *San Yin Jiao* (Sp 6), and *Yang Ling Quan* (GB 34)

Treatment method: Needle using draining technique except at *San Yin Jiao* (Sp 6) which should be supplemented.

Explanation of the formula: Selection of the sea point of the hand *yang ming*, *Qu Chi* (LI 11), in combination with *He Gu* (LI 4) is intended to resolve the exterior and dispel wind. Besides, since the skin is governed by the lungs, these two points on the large intestine channel, which has an exterior-interior relationship with the lungs, may free the lung qi. Fortifying the spleen through *San Yin Jiao* (Sp 6) is expected to transform and move dampness. *Xue Hai* (Sp 10) harmonizes the blood, while *Yang Ling Quan* (GB 34) is an effective point for soothing the sinews and quickening the network vessels.

2. Kidney yang insufficiency pattern: This pattern is established if there are the complications of low back soreness, ringing in the ears, aversion to cold, chilled limbs, a pale facial complexion, loose stools, long voidings of clear urine, menstural irregularity in women, and seminal emission in men. The pulse is fine and bowstring, and the tongue is pale with white fur.

Treatment principles: Warm and supplement kidney yang, secure the defensive and harmonize the constructive

Formula: *Shen Shu* (Bl 23), *Ming Men* (GV 4), and *Zu San Li* (St 36)

Treatment method: Needle using supplementing technique and then moxa.

Explanation of the formula: *Shen Shu* (Bl 23) directly connects with the kidneys, while *Ming Men* (GV 4) is the gate of the source qi or prenatal qi which is stored in the kidneys. The combination of these two is able to greatly boost kidney yang and supplement the kidneys. *San Li* (St 36) is intended to harmonize the qi and blood, secure the defensive and harmonize the constructive.

Note: There is a sub-pattern with invading cold evils which is characterized by purple-colored, chilled hands and feet exacerbated by cold, occasional pain in the affected joints, hair loss, and absence of sweat. The pulse is tight and bowstring. The formula is composed of *Qu Chi* (LI 11), *He Gu* (LI 4), *San Li* (St 36), and *Tai Chong* (Liv 3). These points are punctured with supplementing hand technique with the needles being heated by mugwort burnt on the heads of the needles during retention.

3. Blood stasis pattern: The characteristics of this pattern include purple-colored, chilled extremities, a dull, somber facial complexion, purplish lips, a dry mouth but no desire to drink, menstrual irregularity, a dark purplish tongue with possible static spots or macules, and a fine, choppy pulse. This pattern mainly involves the limbs.

Treatment principles: Quicken the blood and transform stasis, free the flow of the channels and quicken the network vessels

Formula: *Jian Yu* (LI 15), *Qu Chi* (LI 11), *Wai Guan* (TB 5), *He Gu* (LI 4), *San Li* (St 36), *Yin Ling Quan* (Sp 9), *San Yin Jiao* (Sp 6), and *Tai Chong* (Liv 3)

Treatment method: Needle all the above points using draining technique.

Explanation of the formula: To move stasis, it is necessary to free the circulation of the qi and blood. The peculiarity of this team is the selection of pertinent points on both the upper and lower limbs to free the qi and quicken the blood throughout the body. *San Yin Jiao* (Sp 6) and *Yin Ling Quan* (Sp 9) are intended to harmonize the blood while also fortifying the spleen and, thereby, the central qi. *Tai Chong* (Liv 3) is the source point of the liver and hence is a miraculous point for normalizing of the blood and freeing the flow of the network vessels. *He Gu* (LI 4), *Qu Chi* (LI 11), etc. are able to boost the qi.

4. Lung-involving enduring pattern: If skin impediment persists for a long time, it will debilitate the defensive. Since the defensive is weak, wind cold may easily invade the lungs. In consequence, coughing, thin, white phlegm, a cold body, aversion to cold, and, in severe cases, dyspneic breathing with rales, chest oppression, and shortness of breath may occur. The tongue fur is white and glossy, and the pulse is tight.

Treatment principles: Diffuse the lungs and transform phlegm

Formula: *Feng Men* (Bl 12), *Fei Shu* (Bl 13), *Shan Zhong* (CV 17), *Kong Zui* (Lu 6), and *Feng Long* (St 40)

Treatment method: Needle using draining technique.

Explanation of the formula: *Fei Shu* (Bl 13), the transporting point of the lung channel qi, helps diffuse the lungs, and, together with *Shan Zhong* (CV 17), normalizes and courses the qi. According to the classical explanation, *Kong Zui* (Lu 6), the cleft point of the lungs, is a point able to downbear and rectify the lung qi. Together with *San Li* (St 36), *Feng Long* (St 40) transforms phlegm.

5. Chest yang blockage & stagnation pattern: This pattern is indicated by the complications of chest fullness and oppression, purple-colored, chilled extremities, and a dark red tongue body. The pulse is fine and weak.

Treatment principles: Diffuse blockage and free the flow of chest yang, quicken the blood and transform stasis

Formula: *Xin Shu* (Bl 15), *Du Shu* (Bl 16), *Jue Yin Shu* (Bl 14), *Ge Shu* (Bl 17), *Nei Guan* (Per 6), *Shen Men* (Ht 7), *Qu Chi* (LI 11), and *San Li* (St 36)

Explanation of the formula: The back transporting points can free yang and quicken the circulation of the qi to move and transform stasis and disinhibit blockage. *Nei Guan* (Per 6) and *Shen Men* (Ht 7) are needled to free the heart vessel, quicken the blood, and transform stasis. *Qu Chi* (LI 11) and *San Li* (St 36) course the channel qi in the upper and lower body and harmonize the qi and blood in order to remove stagnation and stasis.

6. Spleen & stomach vacuity pattern: As always is the case with spleen-stomach vacuity weakness, this pattern manifests a sallow yellow facial complexion, fatigue, torpid intake, oppression and fullness in the stomach duct or epigastrium, abdominal distention, loose stools, and a weak, soggy pulse. The tongue is pale with white fur.

Treatment principles: Fortify the spleen and harmonize the stomach

Formula: *Pi Shu* (Bl 20), *Wei Shu* (Bl 21), *San Li* (St 36), *Yin Ling Quan* (Sp 9), and *He Gu* (LI 4)

Treatment method: Needle using supplementing technique.

Other choices:

1. Press or puncture the auricular points Endocrine (MA), Liver (MA-SC5), Spleen (MA), and Lung (MA-IC1).

2. Tap the affected part with a cutaneous needle until the skin becomes red.

References:

There is a study on treatment of scleroderma by moxibustion. There were 21 cases studied, of which 6 were localized and 15 were systemic. Moxibustion was applied over medicinal cakes which were prepared from Radix Aconiti Coreani (*Bai Fu Zi*), Resina Olibani (*Ru Xiang*), Resina Myrrhae (*Mo Yao*), Flos Caryophylli (*Ding Xiang*), Herba Asari Cum Radice (*Xi Xin*), Fructus Foeniculi Vulgaris (*Hui Xiang*), Rhizoma Atractylodis (*Cang Zhu*), and Radix Lateralis Praeparatus Aconiti Carmichaeli (*Fu Zi*). The following four groups of points were moxaed by turn directly with cones or with a moxa roll or over the medicated cake: a) *Da Zhui* (GV 14) and *Shen Shu* (BL 23); b) *Ming Men* (GV 4) and *Pi Shu* (Bl 20); c) *Qi Hai* (CV 6) and *Xue Hai* (Sp 10); d) *Ge Shu* (Bl 17) and *Fei Shu* (Bl 13). Moxibustion was performed 2 times per week. During this treatment, all other therapies including Chinese medicinals were suspended. The results were 12 successes. Gui Jin-shui: *Shang Hai Zhen Jiu Za Zhi (Shanghai J. of Acu. & Mox.)* 1980; (1).

There is another report on 1 case of scleroderma treated by moxaing in a similar way as above. The points moxaed included *Qu Chi* (LI 11), *San Li* (St 36), *San Yin Jiao* (Sp 6), *Xue Hai* (Sp 10), *Yang Chi* (TB 4), *Zhong Wan* (CV 12), *Guan Yuan* (CV 4), *Da Zhui* (GV 14), *Shen Shu* (Bl 23),

Ming Men (GV 4), *Pi Shu* (Bl 20), and *Gao Huang Shu* (Bl 43). Four months of treatment cured the case. Wu Jia-qing: *Fu Jian Zhong Yi Za Zhi (Fujian J. of C.M.)* 1984; 15(2):25.

There is another report of 2 cases of localized scleroderma treated by the combination of needle-implanting and moxibustion. One needle was embedded lengthwise on either side of the lesion and changed 1 time every 3 days. The lesion was also moxaed. Two months of treatment cured both cases. Zhong Ji-shang: *Zhe Jiang Zhong Yi Za Zhi (Zhejiang J. of C.M.)* 1986; 21(2):66.

6
Sinew Impediment (Myotenositis Musculi Supraspinati) (1)

This disease is included under exposed shoulder wind in some old classics. It is a pain in the outer side of the shoulder which may extend to the arm or even the fingers. The distinctive feature of this disease is noticeable exacerbation of the pain with abduction of the arm up to a 60° angle. Beyond that degree, the pain quickly and markedly decreases.

Disease causes, disease mechanisms

This disease is due to taxation of the arm and shoulder and invasion of wind cold or cold dampness.

Treatment principles: Harmonize the blood and free the flow of the network vessels, soothe the sinews and stop pain

Formula: *Jian Liao* (TB 14), *Ju Gu* (LI 16), *Nao Shu* (SI 10), *Wai Guan* (TB 5), and *Qu Chi* (LI 11)

Treatment method: Puncture using draining technique, the needle in *Jian Liao* (TB 14) being heated by burning mugwort on its head during retention.

Explanation of the formula: The shoulder and area around the scapula are abundant in "wind holes." Therefore, they are subject to invasion of external evils and especially wind. These invading evils are yang in nature and cause a repletion pattern. This situation makes it necessary to drain the pertinent points on the yang channels of the hand.

Other choices:

1. Press or puncture the auricular points Shoulder (MA-SF4), Endocrine (MA), and Spirit Gate (MA-TF1).

2. Tap the affected area with a cutaneous needle until the skin becomes red.

3. Break the subcutaneous fiber(s) at the tender point(s) with a three-edged needle and then moxa over them.

Case history: A male, aged 46, suffered from pain in his shoulder and upper back. The case was diagnosed as myotenositis musculi supraspinati for which he had received block therapy and medication to no avail. I pressed at the auricular points Shoulder (MA-SF4), Nape, and Spirit Gate (MA-TF1). One treatment relieved the pain.

7
Sinew Impediment (Rhomboideus Strain) (2)

This is also a pain in the shoulder and upper back, usually on one side only. The pain may involve the neck, particularly the back of the neck, which is difficult to turn or bend. Tender points are located along the medial side of the scapula. When caused by sprain, this disease is characterized by its sudden onset.

Treatment principles: Soothe the sinews and quicken the network vessels, dispel wind and scatter cold

Formula: *Da Zhui* (GV 14), *Feng Chi* (GB 20), *Jian Wai Shu* (SI 14), *Kun Lun* (Bl 60), *Hou Xi* (SI 3), and *a shi* points

Treatment method: Needle using draining technique except for the *a shi* points. These should be moxaed or punctured with the needle being warmed by mugwort burnt on the head of the needle during retention.

Explanation of the formula: Because this disease mainly affects the governing vessel and foot *tai yang* channel, *Da Zhui* (GV 14), the meeting point of all the yang channels, is indispensable for dispelling wind and scattering cold as well as freeing the channel qi. *Kun Lun* (Bl 60) is able to course the foot *tai yang* channel to free the channel and its network vessels. *Feng Chi* (Wind Pool, GB 20), as its name suggests, is good at dispelling wind. *Hou Xi* (SI 3) is a point which has proven specific for pain in the back, both the upper and lower back. In addition, *Kun Lun* and *Hou Xi* are among the choices for soothing the sinews.

Other choices:

1. Perform sliding cupping over the affected area.

2. Electroacupuncture the two teams: a) *Jian Wai Shu* (SI 14) and *Hou Xi* (SI 3) and b) *Da Zhu* (Bl 11) and *Kun Lun* (Bl 60).

3. Perform cutaneous needling on the affected part until the skin becomes red and then cup over it.

Case history: A male factory worker, aged 51, underwent chest surgery and two months later suffered from aching and pain in his shoulder and upper back. This was worse when the chest was thrown out. A tender point was found a little above the spina scapulae, and it was moxaed over ginger. Five treatments relieved much of the pain. Ten treatments and the patient recovered.

Reference: There is a report on 256 cases of rhomboideus strain treated by acupuncture. The techniques included cutaneous needling along three lines, a) 0.5 *fen* bilateral to the spine from the 1st thoracic to the 12th thoracic vertebra, b) from *Da Zhu* (Bl 11) to *Ge Shu* (Bl 17), and c) from *Fu Fen* (Bl 41) to *Ge Guan* (Bl 46). Then 1-2 local tender points were punctured with the needle(s) first inserted at an angle of about 75 degrees to a shallow depth. These were then pushed deeper until they were at a right angle to the skin. At that point, the patient might feel an aching or distended sensation at the point(s). Then lifting and thrusting needle manipulation was performed. In the process, a clicking sound might be heard at the needled point(s). This is the sound of subcutaneous fiber(s) severing. After extraction of the needle(s), a bit of blood was pressed out from the hole(s). Of all the cases in the study, 236 were healed; 14 showed marked improvement; and 6 showed some effect. Yang Yi-zhong: *Zhong Guo Zhen Jiu (Chin. Acu. & Mox.)* 1995; (2):7.

8
Neck & Shoulder Pain (Cervical Spondylosis)

Cervical spondylosis may be complicated by many different disorders, such as dizziness and headache. Some complications may overshadow it in severity. Accordingly, in the old medical classics, it was not always categorized as an independent pattern but was sometimes described as a complication of, for instance, *bi*, wilting, and headache.

Disease causes, disease mechanisms

The main site of disease is the back of the neck. Therefore, it is ascribed to the governing vessel and foot *tai yang* channel. Stagnant qi and blood is directly responsible for this disease. This stagnation is, in turn, a product of inhibition of the channels and network vessels due to liver-kidney vacuity and/or invasion of external evils. Since the elderly are liable to depletion of the liver and kidneys, they are the group most likely to contract this kind of disorder.

Treatment based on pattern discrimination

There are four patterns of neck and shoulder pain:

1. Impediment pattern: This type is characterized by stiffness and pain in the neck which may extend to the forearm, the hand, and even the fingers, the tips of which may feel numb. Movement of the shoulder may be limited. The condition gets worse at night.

2. Wilting pattern: This pattern often manifests as discomfort in the neck which is unable to stretch. There is pain in the neck and shoulder with heavy, numb limbs. In severe cases, spasmodic paralysis and fecal and urinary incontinence may develop.

3. Dizziness pattern: This pattern is distinguished by dizziness, headache, ringing in the ears, and numbness of the extremities. In severe cases, there may be sudden collapse.

4. Impaired sense organ pattern: This pattern is peculiar for its distended sensation in the eyes, impaired vision, ringing in the ears or deafness, blockage of the throat, heart palpitations, insomnia, profuse dreaming, and numbness of the hands.

Furthermore, this disease should be analysed in terms of its cause. If it is caused by inhibition of the *tai yang* channel, such signs and symptoms as headache, aversion to cold, stiffness of the whole body, and top-heaviness may manifest. If it is due to liver-kidney vacuity, weak and aching knees and low back, impotence, dizziness, and wilting may manifest.

Treatment principles: Dispel wind and scatter cold, soothe the sinews and quicken the network vessels, disinhibit the qi and stop pain

Formula 1: *Feng Fu* (GV 16), *Da Zhui* (GV 14), *Tian Zhu* (Bl 10), *Da Zhu* (Bl 11), *Feng Chi* (GB 20), *Jian Jing* (GB 21), *Tian Liao* (TB 15), *Tian Zong* (SI 11), local *a shi* points, *Luo Zhen* (M-UE-24), and the cervical *Hua Tuo Jia Ji* points

Modifications: If the focus is located on the route of the governing vessel, it is necessary to choose *Da Zhui* (GV 14), *Tao Dao* (GV 13), *Feng Fu* (GV 16), and *Gu Shu* (Bl 16). If the focus is located on the route of the *tai yang* channel, it is necessary to choose *Tian Zhu* (Bl 10), *Da Zhu* (Bl 11), *Jian Zhong Shu* (SI 15), *Jian Wai Shu* (SI 16), and *Kun Lun* (Bl 60). If the focus is located on the route of the hand *yang ming* channel, it is necessary to include *Qu Chi* (LI 11) and *Shou San Li* (LI 10). If the focus is located on the route of the *shao yang* channel, it is necessary to include *Tian Jing* (TB 10), *Zhi Gou* (TB 6), *Xuan Zhong* (GB 39), and *Qiu Xu* (GB 40). For an inhibited *tai yang* channel pattern with exterior manifestations, add *He Gu* (LI 4), *Lie Que* (Lu 7), *Tai Yang* (M-HN-9), *Shang Xing* (GV 23), and *Yin Tang* (M-HN-3).

For an impediment pattern with severe numbness, add *Jian Yu* (LI 15) and *Qu Chi* (LI 11). If the numbness reaches the tips of the fingers, add *He Gu* (LI 4). In case of headache, add *Feng Chi* (GB 20) and *Bai Hui* (GV 20). In case of pain in the low back and legs, add *Yao Shu* (GV 2), *Ming Men* (GV 4), *Shen Shu* (Bl 23), *Wei Zhong* (Bl 40), and *Yao Yang Guan* (GV 3). In case of liver-kidney vacuity, add *Shen Shu* (Bl 23), *Gan Shu* (Bl 18), *Qi Hai* (CV 6), and *San Li* (St 36).

Treatment method: In each treatment, needle 3-7 points using lifting and thrusting method, supplementing or draining depending upon vacuity or repletion. One can moxa the cervical points which may achieve a better result.

Explanation of the formula: *Luo Zhen* (M-UE-24) is often an indispensable point because it has proven effective for lesions in the soft tissues of the neck. Clinical evidence shows that it can adjust the qi of the three hand yang channels. It frees the flow to the head. And it relaxes and relieves hypertonicity of the muscles of the neck. *Da Zhui* (GV 14) is the point where all the yang channels meet and hence is able to free the flow of qi of all the yang channels and further quicken the blood. *Feng Fu* (GV 16) and *Feng Chi* (GB 20) dispel wind and scatter cold. *Da Zhu* (Bl 11) is the meeting point of the bones and is able to drain heat and relieve pain in the shoulder, upper back, and back of the neck. *Tian Zong* (SI 11), *Jian Zhong Shu* (SI 15), and *Jian Wai Shu* (SI 16) are wonderful points for treating troubles in the shoulder, back of the neck, and upper back.

Formula 2: a) *Feng Chi* (GB 20) and *Kun Lun* (Bl 60); b) *Tian Zhu* (Bl 10) and *Xuan Zhong* (GB 39); c) *Hou Xi* (SI 3) and *Da Zhu* (Bl 11)

Treatment method: Needle the above three groups alternately, using 1 group each treatment.

Modifications: Add *Wai Guan* (TB 5) and the *Shi Xuan* (M-UE-1-5) for an impediment pattern, *i.e.*, numbness in the fingers. Add *Shuai Gu* (GB 8) in case of dizziness. Add *Zhao Hai* (Ki 6) and *Ming Men* (GV 4) in case of kidney vacuity. Add *Nei Guan* (Per 6) in case of chest oppression, nausea, and heart fluster. Add *Xin Shu* (Bl 15) in case of insomnia. Add *Feng Fu* (GV 16) in case of severe dizziness and headache.

Other choices:

1. Moxa the following two groups by turn: a) *Da Zhui* (GV 14) or *Da Zhu* (Bl 11), *Gan Shu* (Bl 18), and *Shen Shu* (Bl 23); b) *Bai Hui* (GV 20) and *Ming Men* (GV 4).

2. Perform cutaneous needling and then cupping at *Da Zhu* (Bl 11), *Tian Zong* (SI 11), *Jian Zhong Shu* (SI 15), and *Jian Wai Shu* (SI 14).

3. Perform warm needling at a point 5 *fen* lateral to the affected cervical vertebra, alternating the point on the two sides. The auxiliary points are *Jian Yu* (LI 15), *Yang Chi* (TB 4), *Tian Zong* (SI 11), and *Qu Chi* (LI 11). Burn 2-3 cones of moxa on the head of the needle for the *a shi* point and 1 cone on each of the auxiliary points. Treat 1 time each day with 7 treatments equalling 1 course.

4. Electroacupuncture the *a shi* point(s) and cervical *Hua Tuo Jia Ji* points as the ruling points plus *Tian Zhu* (Bl 10), *Feng Chi* (GB 20), *Da Zhu* (Bl 11), *Da Zhui* (GV 14), *Qu Chi* (LI 11), *Wai Guan* (TB 5) and *He Gu* (LI 4), using 3-4 points in 1 treatment. Adjust the electric power to the maximum degree that the patient can bear.

5. Puncture or press the auricular points Cervical Vertebra (MA-AH8), Adrenal (MA), and Endocrine (MA-IC3).

6. Prick and then perform cupping at the local *a shi* point(s), *Tian Zong* (SI 11), and *Jian Zhen* (SI 9). After that, massage the affected area while the patient is asked to turn their head about. The massage therapy manipulations include rubbing, pressing, rolling, rocking, and stretching. First, repeatedly rub and press with the thumb from *Feng Fu* (GV 16) through *Ya Men* (GV 15) to *Da Zhui* (GV14). Then do this at *Tian Zhu* (Bl 10) and *Da Zhu* (Bl 11). Continue the same manipulation along the line of *Jian Zhong Shu* (SI 15), *Jian Wai Shu* (SI 14), and *Tian Zong* (SI 11) which is usually a tender place. Then perform rolling along the hand *tai yang* and *yang ming* channels on the arm. Finally, stretch the neck and turn the head with a gentle force. It is better if one applies a hot compress after this treatment.

Reference: There is a report on 243 cases of cervical spondylosis treated by acupuncture in combination with massage therapy. The ruling points used were *Feng Chi* (GB 20) and cervical *Hua Tuo Jia Ji* points, and the auxiliary points were *Jian Zhen* (SI 9), *Jian Yu* (LI 15), *Bi Nao* (LI 14), *Qu Chi* (LI 11), *Shou San Li* (LI 10), *Wai Guan* (TB 5), and *He Gu* (LI 4). In each treatment, 4 ruling points and 3 supplemental points were chosen. For the ruling points, there was no need to retain the needles. All the auxiliary points were used unilaterally. In other words, only those located on the affected side were needled. For them, needle retention was required. After extraction of the needles, the patient was made to sit straight to receive a combination of manipulations including rubbing, pressing, rolling, and pinching the back of the neck. Then the practitioner pressed the tender point(s) for 5 minutes. In case of a deviated spinous process, the practitioner might perform joint reduction and then pulling apart at *Jian Jing* (GB 21). One hundred four cases were completely cured; 113 reported improvement; and 26 showed no effect. The total effectiveness rate was 89%. Luo Yan: *Zhong Guo Zhen Jiu (Chin. Acu. & Mox.)* 1995; (5):14.

9
Articular Wind (Rheumatic Arthritis)

The literal meaning of the Chinese term, *li jie feng*, is wind visiting the joints, and its other name is wind dampness disease (*feng shi bing*). This tells us that this disease is migratory or progressive in nature, visiting from joint to joint, and that its main disease causes are wind and dampness. This is the disease category most often directly mentioned by the term impediment. If the knee is swollen, painful, and hot, this is called crane's knee wind. Articular wind may be menacing, for it not only produces swelling and pain in the related joints but causes permanent lesions to them, thus restricting their movement.

Treatment based on pattern discrimination

This disease is classified into two patterns: the wind, cold, and dampness pattern and the wind, dampness, and heat pattern. The first pattern is characterized by aching in the muscles around the affected joint which is worse in wet weather. The second pattern manifests hot signs and symptoms. Each of these two patterns, however, may be further divided into a number of sub-patterns according to the different evils predominating in them.

1. Migratory impediment pattern: Wind is the principal culprit. There is pain in the joints which is migratory, not fixed to any one joint, but moving from one to another. There is also possible fever, aversion to cold, white or slimy tongue fur, and a floating pulse.

Treatment principles: Dispel wind and free the flow of the network vessels, scatter cold and eliminate dampness

Formula: *Feng Chi* (GB 20), *Ge Shu* (Bl 17), *Xue Hai* (Sp 10), and *Tai Chong* (Liv 3)

Treatment method: Needle using twirling drainage.

Explanation of the formula: *Feng Chi* (GB 20) resolves the exterior and courses wind. *Xue Hai* (Sp 10) and *Ge Shu* (Bl 17) are intended to quicken the blood with the implication that once blood is moved, wind will die down by itself. *Tai Chong* (Liv 3) rectifies the qi to quicken the blood.

2. Painful impediment pattern: This pattern is characterized by pain which is intense and fixed, getting better when it receives heat but getting worse with cold. The principal culprit is cold. In painful impediment, the local skin is not red and does not feel hot and the tongue fur is white with a floating, tight pulse.

Treatment principles: Warm the channels and scatter cold, dispel wind and eliminate dampness

Formula: *Shen Shu* (Bl 23) and *Guan Yuan* (CV 4)

Treatment method: Needle with even manipulation, *i.e.*, neither supplementing nor draining technique. Needling should be followed by moxibustion each treatment.

Explanation of the formula: This is in fact cold impediment. When cold prevails, yang qi must be debilitated. Therefore, to treat such a case, one should warm and free yang to drive out cold. To accomplish this task, *Shen Shu* (Bl 23) is a most appropriate point because it has direct access to the kidneys where the true yang or life fire is stored. *Guan Yuan* (CV 4) is a well known point for its ability to stimulate the source qi which is the same as the yang qi.

3. Fixed impediment pattern: This pattern, in which dampness predominates, is diagnosed if there is aching and heaviness in the affected joints and muscles or diffuse swelling around the affected joints with fixed pain and insensitivity of the local skin. The pulse is usually soggy and slow.

Treatment principles: Eliminate dampness and free the flow of the network vessels, dispel wind and scatter cold

Formula: *Yin Ling Quan* (Sp 9) and *Zu San Li* (St 36)

Treatment method: Needle using lifting and thrusting supplementation.

Explanation of the formula: Since dampness is the predominant factor in this category, the spleen has to be fortified in order to eliminate it. These two points bank the spleen from both the yin and yang aspects so that the transformation and generation of the spleen may be strengthened.

4. Hot impediment pattern: This pattern is distinguished by its sudden onset, burning heat, and fulminant swelling around the affected joints which gets better when subjected to cold. There is often thirst, vexation and agitation, and fever which persists in spite of copious sweating. The tongue is red with yellow or slimy, yellow fur, and the pulse is rapid and slippery.

Treatment principles: Clear heat and disinhibit dampness, dispel wind and quicken the blood

Formula: *Da Zhui* (GV 14), *Qu Chi* (LI 11), and *He Gu* (LI 4)

Treatment method: Needle using lifting and thrusting drainage except for *Da Zhui* (GV 14) which should be pricked with a three-edged needle. This pricking should be followed by cupping to induce more bleeding.

Explanation of the formula: *Da Zhui* (GV 14) is a wonderful point to clear heat and dispel wind because it has access to the yang qi of the whole body. The other two points, both on the *yang ming* channel which abounds in qi and blood, resolve the exterior, clear heat, and disperse swelling.

5. Stubborn impediment: Besides the above, there is also a pattern known as stubborn impediment which is further separated into two sub-patterns: the cold and the hot.

In the hot stubborn impediment, the joints are swollen with heat and pain, possibly accompanied by tidal fever, vexation, thirst, night sweats, and aversion to wind. There may be red papules or nodules, wasted, emaciated muscles, red or crimson tongue, and a fine, rapid or rapid, bowstring pulse. In cold stubborn impediment, the joints are also swollen and painful but with aversion to cold in the locally affected area. The pain and swelling are worse with cold but better with heat. Bending and stretching of the affected joints are inhibited. There may be a cold body and generalized aversion to wind. The tongue is light or dark red with thin, white fur, and the pulse is deep and slow or fine and bowstring.

Treatment principles: Enrich yin and boost yang, move the qi and quicken the blood, dispel wind and eliminate dampness

Formula: *Qi Hai* (CV 6), *San Yin Jiao* (Sp 6), and *Tai Xi* (Ki 3)

Treatment method: Needle using lifting and thrusting drainage on the first two points and twirling drainage on the last.

Explanation of the formula: *Qi Hai* (CV 6) boosts the qi and secures yang. *San Yin Jiao* (Sp 6) and *Tai Xi* (Ki 3) enrich yin and clear heat through supplementing and boosting the liver and spleen.

All of the above discussions concern the elimination of the root of the disease causes of the various types of impediment. However, in the treatment of impediment, one must also give adequate attention to the selection of local points in accordance with the affected channels. Below is a list of frequently used local points:

For the jaw joint, choose *Xia Guan* (St 7), *Yin Feng* (TB 17), and *He Gu* (LI 4).

For cervical joints, choose *Feng Chi* (GB 20), *Wan Gu* (GB 12), and *Tian Zhu* (Bl 10).

For thoracic vertebral joints, choose *Hua Tuo Jia Ji* points which are located 5 *fen* bilateral to the spine.

For sacrococcygeal joints, choose *Da Chang Shu* (Bl 25), *Ming Men* (GV 4), *Ba Liao* (Bl 31-34), and *Wei Zhong* (Bl 40).

For the shoulder joints, choose *Jian Yu* (LI 15), *Tian Zong* (SI 11), and *Ji Quan* (Ht 1).

For the elbow joint, choose *Qu Chi* (LI 11), *Xiao Hai* (SI 8), *Zhou Liao* (LI 12), and *Shou San Li* (LI 10).

For the wrist joints, choose *Wai Guan* (TB 5), *Yang Chi* (TB 4), and *Wan Gu* (SI 4).

For the phalangeal and metacarpal joints, choose the *Ba Xie* (M-UE-22), *He Gu* (LI 4), and *Hou Xi* (SI 3).

For the iliac joint, choose *Guan Yuan Shu* (Bl 26), *Xiao Chang Shu* (Bl 27), *Bai Huan Shu* (Bl 30), *Huan Tiao* (GB 30), *Zhi Bian* (Bl 54), and *Ju Liao* (GB 29).

For the hip joint, choose *Huan Tiao* (GB 30) and *Yang Ling Quan* (GB 34).

For the knee joint, choose *Du Bi* (St 35), *Xi Yan* (M-LE-16a), *Qu Quan* (Liv 8), and *Wei Zhong* (Bl 40).

For the ankle joint, choose *Jie Xi* (St 41), *Shang Qiu* (Sp 5), *Qiu Xu* (GB 40), *Kun Lun* (Bl 60), *Tai Xi* (Ki 3), *Shen Mai* (Bl 62), and *Zhao Hai* (Ki 6).

For the metatarsal and phalangeal joints, choose *Jie Xi* (St 41), *Gong Sun* (Sp 4), *Tai Chong* (Liv 3), *Zu Lin Qi* (GB 41), and the *Ba Feng* (M-LE-8).

Other choices:

1. Moxibustion: Ruling points: *A shi* points, *Da Zhui* (GV 14), *Jian Yu* (LI 15), *Qu Chi* (LI 11), *He Gu* (LI 4), *Feng Shi* (GB 31), *San Yin Jiao* (Sp 6), *Jue Gu* (GB 39), *Shen Zhu* (GV 12), *Yao Yang Guan* (GV 3), *Shen Shu* (Bl 23), and *Qi Hai* (CV 6). Auxiliary points: *Xia Guan* (St 7), *Ting Gong* (SI 19), and *Yi Feng* (TB 17) for the jaw joint. The *Ba Xie* (M-UE-22) and *Si Feng* (M-UE-9) for the phalangeal joints. *Yang Chi* (TB 4), *Da Ling* (Per 7), *Yang Xi* (LI 5), and *Wan Gu* (SI 4) for the wrist joint. *Tian Jing* (TB 10) and *Qu Ze* (Per 3) for the elbow joint. *Jian Yu* (LI 15) and *Jian Zhen* (SI 9) for the shoulder joint. *Ming Men* (GV 4) and the corresponding *Hua Tuo Jia Ji* points for the vertebral joints. The points below the seventeenth vertebra, and *Bai Huan Shu* (Bl 30) for the sacrococcygeal joints. *Xiao Chang Shu* (Bl 27) and *Pang Guang Shu* (Bl 28) for the iliac joints. *Huan Tiao* (GB 30) and *Ju Liao* (GB 29) for the hip joint. *Xi Yan* (M-LE-16a),

Yin Ling Quan (Sp 9) and *Yang Ling Quan* (GB 34) for the knee joint. *Kun Lun* (Bl 60), *Jie Xi* (St 41), *Tai Xi* (Ki 3), and *Qiu Xu* (GB 40) for the ankle joint. And the *Ba Feng* (M-LE-8) and *Shang Qiu* (Sp 5) for metatarsal and phalangeal joints. Choose 2-4 points from the above each treatment.

2. Electroacupuncture: Ruling points: *Huan Tiao* (GB 30), *Yang Ling Quan* (GB 34), *Xuan Zhong* (GB 39), *He Gu* (LI 4), *Qu Chi* (LI 11), *Da Zhui* (GV 14), and *Jian Yu* (LI 15). Auxiliary points: *Bi Nao* (LI 14), *Jian Shi* (Per 5), *Shao Hai* (Ht 3), *San Li* (St 36), *Wei Zhong* (Bl 40), *Kun Lun* (Bl 60), and *Jie Xi* (St 42). After inserting the needles, the electric current should be increased little by little to the maximum that the patient can stand.

Case history: A female, aged 53, complained of tubercles in her thigh which never failed to recur every spring for many years. These tubercles were hard and painful and the areas around them were swollen. There was pain in the joints of the lower limbs. Flash moxibustion was prescribed. The moxibustion was performed at the center of every tubercle with a thin burning moxa roll which was put on the point and quickly put out by being pressed against the skin. Following this, the pain in the tubercles disappeared and the pain in the joints was relieved to some degree. Two months later, however, two tubercles reappeared. The same technique was used again, and the tubercles were gone for good.

Reference: There is a report on the different effects on two groups brought by needling alone and by needling in combination with cupping. The points chosen included local and distant points, but the ruling ones were *a shi* points. In case of shoulder arthritis, *Jian Yu* (LI 15), *Jian Liao* (TB 14), *Jian Jing* (GB 21), and *Tian Zong* (SI 11) were included. For elbow arthritis, *Qu chi* (LI 11), *Tian Jing* (TB 10), and *Shou San Li* (LI 10) were included. In case of lumbar and iliac arthritis, *Yao Yang Guan* (GV 3), *Guan Yuan Shu* (Bl 26), *Xiao Chang Shu* (Bl 27), *Pang Guang Shu* (Bl 28), *Zhi Bian* (Bl 54), and *Huan Tiao* (GB 30) were included. In case of knee arthritis, *Liang Qiu* (St 34), *Xue Hai* (Sp 10), *Xi Yang Guan* (GB 33), *Qu Quan* (Liv 8), *Wai Xi Yan* (St 35), *Nei Xi Yan* (M-LE-16a), and *Zu San Li* (St 36) were included. In case of ankle arthritis, *Jue Gu* (GB 39), *Tai Xi* (Ki 3), and *Kun Lun* (Bl 60) were included. The combined therapy was described as follows: After insertion, the needles were twirled to induce the qi and were then retained for 10 minutes. Then the practitioner twirled the needles again to keep up the stimulation and, with the needles in position, performed cupping over the needled points. The cupping continued for about 10 minutes. Finally, the cups were removed and the needles were twirled once more before they were extracted. Three hundred cases of arthritis were treated by means of combined needling and cupping. One hundred twenty-eight recovered; 81 reported noticeable effect; 66 showed improvement; and 25 had no response. The total effectiveness rate in the combined therapy group was 91.67%. The control group, which also consisted of 300 cases of arthritis, was treated by simple needling. Of these, 57 were healed; 78 showed marked improvement; and 102 got some effect. The total effectiveness rate in this group was 79%. Sun Jing-de: *Zhong Guo Zhen Jiu (Chin. Acu. & Mox.),* 1986; (6):7.

10
Deformation Impediment (Rheumatoid Arthritis)

This disease is also been called bone *bi* and damp heat *bi* in the old medical classics.

Disease causes, disease mechanisms

In most cases, the patient is weak with qi and blood insufficiency. Because their righteous qi is depleted, when cold and dampness evils invade, they may settle deep, blocking the channels and network vessels. Since the vessels are inhibited, dampness gathers into phlegm which may penetrate the sinews, bones, and joints. Thus there appears wilting, stiffness, and hypertonicity of the sinew vessels and muscles with eventual joint deformation. Thus it is clear that this disease is due to a root vacuity with a replete branch or righteous qi vacuity with evil qi repletion. At its onset, there may be fatigue, weight loss, torpid intake, low-grade fever, and numbness in the extremities. At this time, only the minor joints, for example, the knuckles or the wrists or ankles are involved. With the slow progression of the disease, various major joints will eventually be affected.

Treatment principles: Clear heat and disinhibit dampness, quicken the blood and free the flow of the network vessels

Treatment method: Same as those for articular wind.

Note: The author's clinical experience proves that acupuncture and moxibustion are good for deformation impediment of recent onset. (However,) it takes a long time for any therapy to bring effect. Therefore, she especially uses moxibustion treating this disease, since it can be performed at home by the patient themself or by their relatives after careful instruction. In the advanced stage, acumoxatherapy alone often offers little help. Therefore, it is better to prescribe a combined protocol of acumoxatherapy with some other alternative therapy or therapies. Oral administration of Chinese medicinals may accelerate recovery. In designing a formula of either medication or acumoxatherapy, one should take into consideration which viscus and/or bowel is involved.

References:

There is a report on 150 cases treated with warm needling. The points used were *Shui Gou* (GV 26), *Wei Zhong* (Bl 40), *Ji Quan* (Ht 1), and local points around the affected joint(s). The treatment procedures were to induce the qi after inserting the needles and then burn mugwort cones on the heads of the needles during their retention. In the afternoon, another treatment was given, in which the *Ba Liao* (Bl 31-34) and *Hua Tuo Jia Ji* points were punctured with 20 minutes of needle retention. In the course of treatment, massage therapy, washing and steaming of the affected joints, and oral administration of medicinal formulas were prescribed. The report says that 17 cases were cured; 47 showed noticeable effect; 77 had improvement, and 9 got no effect. Wang Ji-yuan: *Zhong Yi Za Zhi (J. of C.M.)* 1990; (1).

There is another report on 65 cases of rheumatoid arthritis treated by medicated moxibustion. The preparatory procedures were to sprinkle 8g of a mixture of powdered mylabris (*Ban Mao*), Secretio Moschi Moschiferi (*She Xiang*), Flos Caryophylli (*Ding Xiang*), and Cortex Cinnamomi Cassiae (*Rou Gui*) along the spine from *Da Zhui* (GV 14) to *Yao Shu* (GV 2). A strip of garlic mash 5mm wide and 2.5mm high was then spread over this powder. On top of the layer of garlic, there was another strip of mugwort 3mm wide and 2.5mm high. Then the two ends and the middle of this mugwort strip were lighted. This moxibustion produced blisters which were pricked and dressed with disinfectant 3 days later. Luo Shi-rong: *Zhe Jiang Zhong Yi Za Zhi (Zhejiang J. of C.M.)* 1985; (7):20.

11
Thigh Wind (Piriformis Syndrome)

This is a lancinating or burning pain deep in the hip which radiates along the lateral posterior aspect of the thigh and lower leg. In severe cases, it may even involve the testicles. It may also get worse with urination, defecation, or coughing.

Disease causes, disease mechanisms

This disease is usually caused by contusion and wrenching which damages the muscles of the hip.

Treatment principles: Quicken the blood and free the flow of the network vessels, transform stasis and stop pain

Formula: *Zhi Bian* (Bl 54) and *Wei Zhong* (Bl 40)

Treatment method: Puncture both of these points, retaining the needles for 15 minutes and making sure that the needle qi reaches down to the lower leg. These two points may also be moxaed or electroacupunctured to achieve a similar effect. If moxibustion is used, some pertinent local points may be added.

Other choice: Prick the tender point(s) and then perform cupping over them 2 times each week.

Reference: There is a report on treatment of acute piriformis syndrome. The treatment procedures were as follows: After determining the tenderest point at the piriformis on the hip, a long needle was inserted deep to its focus. This was then lifted and thrust repeatedly in a large amplitude to induce strong stimulation. After that, the needle was withdrawn under the skin and then thrust deeply in opposite directions at 45° angles. Tian Deng-shan: *Zhong Guo Zhen Jiu (Chin. Acu. & Mox.)* 1993; (5): 22.

12
Chest & Rib-side Pain (Costal Chondritis)

This disease appears in the old medical classics as bone impediment.

Treatment based on pattern discrimination

This disease may be caused by coughing or traumatic injury to the ribs or ligaments. Besides pain, there may be chest oppression and distention.

Treatment principles: Move the qi and quicken the blood, free the flow of the network vessels and scatter nodulation

Formula: *Shan Zhong* (CV 17), *Nei Guan* (Per 6), and local *a shi* point(s)

Treatment method: Needle, moxa, or combine needling and moxibustion. When puncturing the local *a shi* points, insert the needles parallel to the sternum or the ribs. Moxibustion can be done over ginger.

Explanation of the formula: There is an old saying, "For any chest and costal (disorders), appeal to *Nei Guan*." From this we can see that *Nei Guan* (Per 6) is an indispensable point in this case. *Shan Zhong* (CV 17) is chosen because it is not only a point adjacent to the trouble but because it is also good at freeing the flow of qi.

Other choices:

1. Perform cutaneous needling on the affected area until the skin becomes red.

2. Press or puncture the auricular points Chest (MA-AH11), Liver (MA-SC5), Spirit Gate (MA-TF1), and Adrenal (MA).

3. Apply powdered Semen Raphani Sativi (*Lai Fu Zi*) on the local *a shi* points. This powder should be fixed in place with an adhesive plaster to keep it from falling off. Change this every day.

Reference: I have treated tens of cases of costal chondritis with the combined needling and moxibustion method instructed above. My total effectiveness rate is 92%. Forty percent were healed completely.

13
Mandibular Pain (Temporomandibular Joint Syndrome)

This disease may be very persistent, possibly lasting for over 10 years. It manifests as pain in and restriction of the movement of the jaws. This pain is worsened by opening of the mouth and chewing.

Treatment principles: Soothe the sinews and quicken the network vessels, warm the channels and scatter cold. Treatment should be directed at the *yang ming* channel.

Formula: *Xia Guan* (St 7) or *San Li* (St 36)

Treatment method: Either warm needling or simple moxibustion is OK.

Other choices:

1. Press or puncture the auricular points Lower Jaw (MA), Upper Jaw (MA), and Adrenal (MA).

2. Electroacupuncture *Jia Che* (St 6) and *Xia Guan* (St 7).

3. Massage therapy: First press and rub *Tai Yang* (M-HN-9), *Tou Wei* (St 5), *Xia Guan* (St 7), and *Jia Che* (St 6). Then press down from *Tai Yang* (M-HN-9) to the jaw.

Case history: A female, aged 30, complained of inability to open her mouth for 2 weeks due to pain in her right jaw joint. Warm needling was performed at *Xia Guan* (St 7) on the affected side. Two treatments effected a cure.

Note: For enduring cases where the jaw joint has already been damaged, simple acumoxatherapy can relieve pain to some degree, but it is difficult to cure this condition completely. One should prescribe a combined therapy, for instance, with massage therapy.

References:

There is a report on 5 cases of TMJ treated by moxa roll. The points selected were the local *a shi* points. All the cases were healed. Dong Zhi-ming: *Zhe Jiang Zhong Yi Za Zhi (Zhejiang J. of C.M.)* 1981; (9):417.

In another report of 40 cases treated by warm needling, the points selected were *Ting Gong* (SI 19), *Ting Hui* (GB 2), and *Xia Guan* (St 7). Warm needling consisted of burning mugwort on the heads of the needles during their retention. Thirty-six cases were healed or showed marked effect. The total effectiveness rate was 97.6%. Qin Gao-zhen: *Zhong Yi Za Zhi (J. of C.M.)* 1983; (8):13.

14
Crick in the Neck (Torticollis)

This is a very common disorder manifesting as sudden hypertonicity of one side of the neck. There may be headache and pain in the neck radiating towards the shoulder and upper back.

Disease causes, disease mechanisms

This condition is usually started by invading wind or inappropriate lying position while sleeping.

Treatment principles: Soothe the sinews and dissipate wind cold, harmonize the qi and quicken the blood

Formula: *Hou Xi* (SI 3), *Xuan Zhong* (GB 39), *a shi* points, and *Luo Zhen* (M-HN-27)

Treatment method: The *a shi* point, which is the tenderest place on the neck, can be treated by cupping. Needle the other points. When needling *Hou Xi* (SI 3), the patient should loosely clench their fist and they should be asked to move their neck while the needle is stimulated and retained. In puncturing *Xuan Zhong* (GB 39), the needle should be inserted slanting upwards to induce a needle sensation which extends upwards.

Explanation of the formula: *Hou Xi* (SI 3) is a point where the *tai yang* channel qi pours in and is one of the eight major intersection points communicating with the governing vessel. As such, it is very good at resolving hypertonicity of and pain in the neck. *Xuan Zhong* (GB 39) is a starting point of a major network vessel and the meeting point of the marrow. Therefore, it is able to soothe the sinews and relax the neck. *Luo Zhen* (M-HN-27) is a point which has been specifically proven effective for this disorder. It harmonizes the blood and dissipates wind cold.

Modifications: Add *He Gu* (LI 4) and *Wai Guan* (TB 5) in case of headache and aversion to cold. Add *Qu Yuan* (SI 13) and *Jian Yu* (LI 15) in case of shoulder pain. Add *Da Zhu* (Bl 11) and *Jian Wai Shu* (SI 14) in case of upper back pain.

Other choices:

1. Moxibustion: Ruling points: *A shi* (points), *Feng Chi* (GB 20), *Tian Zhu* (Bl 10), *Da Zhu* (Bl 11), *Da Zhui* (GV 14), and *Jian Zhong Shu* (SI 15). Auxiliary points: *Jian Wai Shu* (SI 14), *Jian Jing* (GB 21), *Jian Yu* (LI 15), *Qu Chi* (LI 11), *Hou Xi* (SI 3), and *Jue Gu* (GB 39). Moxa directly with cones over ginger or with a moxa roll.

2. Massage therapy: First ask the patient to relax the muscles of their neck while moving the neck about. When it is certain that the muscles are relaxed, help the patient turn their neck towards the affected side. Then perform rolling, pressing, pinching, and rubbing at *Feng Chi* (GB 20), *Feng Fu* (GV 16), *Feng Men* (Bl 12), *Da Zhui* (GV 14), *Jian Jing* (GB 21), and *Tian Zong* (SI 11).

Reference: There is a study of treatment of this disorder by needling the single point, *Shou San Li* (LI 10). The treatment procedures were as follows: The patient was made to sit with the elbow on the affected side bent and set level. A needle was inserted at first to a shallow depth, and then, after the elbow was raised, the needle was pushed to 1.5 *cun* deep. Next, lifting and thrusting manipulation was performed for 2-5 minutes. When the needle sensation was induced, the patient was instructed to move their neck with gradually increasing force and amplitude. After that, the arm was put down and the needle was withdrawn to a shallow depth. The patient was asked to continue turning their neck. If the pain still lingered after this operation, the same procedure was repeated. One hundred cases were treated this way. Of these, 92 were cured and 8 showed improvement. Su Jin-hua: *Zhong Guo Zhen Jiu (Chin. Acu. & Mox.)* 1994; (1):22.

Book Six: Anal Diseases

The anus is called the gate of grains or the gate of the *po*, *i.e.*, the corporeal soul. All diseases relating to the anus appeared under the names of hemorrhoids and fistulas in olden times except for a few individual problems, such as prolapse of the rectum, which were given their own names.

Disease causes, disease mechanisms

In treating diseases of the anus, one should first identify their different causes. There are many discussions of anal diseases in the old classics. The *Dan Xi Xin Fa (The Heart of Danxi's Methods)* published in 1347 CE says, "All cases of hemorrhoids are due to vacuity of the root, external damage by wind dampness, and internal brewing of heat toxins." When discussing hemorrhoids, the *Zheng Zhi Yao Jue (Essentials of Patterns & Treatment)* published by Dai Yuan-li of the Ming dynasty says, "Bleeding is due to wind if the discharged blood is clear, to dampness if the blood is a sooty color, and to heat if the blood is bright red." *The Mirror* says, "If there is cracking around the anus with dry, bound stools, there is fire dryness." To sum up these classical illustrations, there are four disease causes as regards diseases of the anus, namely, wind dryness, damp heat, qi vacuity, and blood vacuity.

1
Prolapse of the Rectum

Disease causes, disease mechanisms

The Simple Questions gives an instructive analysis of the causes of prolapse of the rectum by saying:

> Besides, there are women who have given birth to many children. They sustain exhausted force, dry blood, and qi vacuity. Both these women as well as small children who suffer from enduring dysentery may have prolapse of the rectum.

From this passage, it is clear that insufficient qi and blood with qi fallen below is an important factor responsible for prolapse of the rectum. Because it is fallen below, the qi is no longer able to lift up and contract the anus and hence the rectum protrudes. There is, however, another type in which repletion accounts for the trouble. When damp heat is depressed in the rectum causing hemorrhoids, swelling may appear around the anus. If one strains the anus while evacuating stools, the rectum may also protrude.

Treatment principles: Boost the qi to strengthen its uplifting action, clear heat and disinhibit dampness

Formula: *Bai Hui* (GV 20), *Chang Qiang* (GV 1), *Da Chang Shu* (Bl 25), *San Li* (St 36), and *Qi Hai* (CV 6)

Treatment method: Needle using draining technique. It is better yet to perform fire-needling.

Explanation of the formula: *Chang Qiang* (GV 1) is the starting point of the branch network of the governing vessel around the anus and hence is able to contract the anus. *Bai Hui* (GV 20) is the meeting point of the governing vessel and the yang channels. Therefore, it is particularly good at boosting the yang qi and strengthening its function of upbearing and contracting. *Qi Hai* (Sea of Qi, CV 6), as its name suggests, is related to the source qi and hence is able to invigorate yang and supplement the kidneys to uplift the sunken yang qi. *San Li* (St 36), the sea point of the foot *yang ming*, is a point which has proven able to greatly supplement the central qi to upbear that which has fallen.

Other choices:

1. Moxa *Bai Hui* (GV 20), *Chang Qiang* (GV 1), *Shen Que* (CV 8), *Shui Fen* (CV 9), *Qi Hai* (CV 6), and *San Li* (St 36) with a moxa roll or cones over ginger.

2. Moxa *Shen Que* (CV 8) alone over a layer of salt with 5-10 cones, 1 time each day or every other day. One course consists of 5-7 sessions with an intermission of 3-5 days between courses.

3. Triangular moxibustion: The procedures for this moxibustion method are to draw an equilateral triangle the width of the patient's mouth on each side. Place the top angle or vertex at the center of the navel with the side opposite to the vertex placed horizontally (*i.e.*, the base of the triangle should be directly below the navel). Mark the angles of the sides on the skin and then moxa the marked points.

4. Dab smashed Semen Ricini Communis (*Bi Ma Zi*) at *Bai Hui* (GV 20). This layer of castor beans should be left there for 3-4 hours. Apply this paste every day.

5. Steam and wash the anus with a solution of Galla Rhois Chinensis (*Wu Bei Zi*) and Alum (*Ku Fan*) and then bear up the prolapsed rectum in place with one hand. Do this 1 time each day.

Case history: A male, aged 6, had suffered from prolapse of the rectum for over half a year. This had been refractory to medication and other therapies he had received. One treatment of triangular moxibustion affected a complete recovery.

References:

There is a report of 42 cases of prolapse of the rectum in children treated by moxaing *Bai Hui* (GV 20). Thirty cases were cured, 8 showed improvement, and 4 reported no effect. For mild cases, 3-5 treatments were said to be enough to affect recovery. *Zhong Guo Zhen Jiu Ji Cui (A Collection of Outstanding Works of Chinese Acupuncture & Moxibustion)*, Beijing, People's Health & Hygiene Press, 1986.

There is another report of 40 cases of prolapse of the rectum in children treated by injecting Vitamin B into *Chang Qiang* (GV 1) 1 time every other day. Thirty-eight were cured, 1 showed improvement, and 1 had no effect. Liu Ying-jun: *Zhong Guo Zhen Jiu (Chin. Acu. & Mox.)* 1994; (1):16.

2
Hemorrhoids

Disease causes, disease mechanisms

The Inner Classic says, "Intestinal afflux due to overeating with dilation of the sinew vessels (around the anus) results in hemorrhoids." Based upon this original understanding, later Chinese medical practitioners have been accruing knowledge of this disease and have accumulated rich experience in treating it. From the point of view of Chinese medicine, hemorrhoids are due to accumulated damp heat in the large intestine which produces turbid qi and blood stasis, damaging the channels and network vessels around the anus. This damp heat may, in turn, be a product of undisciplined diet, for instance, eating too much acrid or hot food. Hemorrhoids may also be due to sitting too long, constant constipation, or enduring dysentery or diarrhea.

Treatment principles: Clear heat and disinhibit dampness, quicken the blood and transform stasis

Formula: *Chang Qiang* (GV 1), *Hui Yang* (Bl 35), and *Cheng Shan* (Bl 57)

Modifications: Add *Er Bai* (M-UE-29) and *San Yin Jiao* (Sp 6) in case of bleeding. Add *Bai Hui* (GV 20) in case of prolapse of the hemorrhoid. Add *Zhi Gou* (TB 6) and *Zhao Hai* (Ki 6) in case of constipation.

Treatment method: Needle using draining technique with 15-20 minutes of needle retention.

Other choices:

1. Moxibustion: Ruling points: *Bai Hui* (GV 20), *Tao Dao* (GV 15), *Da Chang Shu* (Bl 25), *Yao Shu* (GV 2), *Chang Qiang* (GV 1), *Cheng Shan* (Bl 57), and local tender points. Auxiliary points: *Ming Men* (GV 4), *Yao Yang Guan* (GV 3), *Pi Shu* (Bl 20), *Shen Shu* (Bl 23), *Bai Huan Shu* (Bl 30), *San Li* (St 36), and *San Yin Jiao* (Sp 9). Each treatment, choose 3-4 points from the above list and moxa them with a moxa roll or cones over ginger. The local points should be moxaed a little longer.

2. Sever the subcutaneous fiber(s) with a three-edged needle under the corresponding brown spot(s) found in the sacral region. After that, perform cupping over the pricked place(s).

3. Fire-needling: Heat a thick needle until red-hot over a fire, and then promptly insert it into the center of the hemorrhoid to let out a bit of blackish blood. This method is good for external hemorrhoids.

4. Cutting *Yin Jiao* (*i.e.,* the frenulum): Carefully inspect the inside of the upper lip and see if there is a small, white growth in the neighborhood of *Yin Jiao* (GV 28). If there is, remove it with a knife, and then press out a bit of blood from the cut.

Case histories:

A male, aged 41, had suffered from hemorrhoids for over 5 years, often with bleeding. On examination, a growth 0.5mm in diameter was found a little bit to the left of the ligament on the inside of the upper lip. This growth was cut off. Twelve hours after the operation, the hemafecia decreased, and 2 days later, it stopped altogether.

Another male, aged 15, complained of itching and pain at the anus which restricted his walking. On examination, an external hemorrhoid as large as a soybean was found at the anus. Fire-needling was performed at the hemorrhoid, and drops of blackish blood were let out. One week later, the case was healed.

Note: Removal of any growths is the author's first choice for treating hemorrhoids provided such a growth can be found. This is because this operation is very easy and simple, and, what's more, quite effective without any side effects.

References:

There is a report of 32 cases of incarcerated internal hemorrhoids treated with combined cutaneous needling and cupping. The procedures were a) tapping with a cutaneous needle paravertebrally from the lumbus to the coccyx until there was slight bleeding; and then b) using four cups, performing cupping to let out more blood (the total amount in a treatment was 15-30ml) 1 time every other day. In between 1-5 sessions, 18 cases were relieved; 7 showed marked effect; and 2 reported no improvement. The total effectiveness rate was 93.8%. Zhou Shi-jie: *Zhong Guo Zhen Jiu (Chin. Acu. & Mox.)* 1994; (1): 8.

There is another study of the treatment of hemorrhoids by merely needling *Er Bai* (M-UE-29). The technique was to first insert the needle to the depth of 1 *cun* and then to twirl it 4 times at 5 minute intervals, withdrawing it a little 3 times and pushing it in a little 1 time. Ninety-nine cases were needled this way. Of these, 64 were cured and 35 showed effect. Ding Dao-wu: *Zhong Guo Zhen Jiu (Chin. Acu. & Mox.)* 1985; (1):11.

3
Splitting of the Anus (Anal Fissure)

Disease causes, disease mechanisms

Splitting of the anus is often a direct product of hard, bound stools which, in turn, are ascribed to blood heat and dry intestines.

Treatment principles: Clear heat and moisten dryness to soften the stools

Formula: *Da Chang Shu* (Bl 25), *Tian Shu* (St 25), and local *a shi* point(s)

Treatment method: Needle the first two points using draining technique. Moxa the *a shi* point(s).

Other choices:

1. Needle *Fei Yang* (Bl 58), *Wei Zhong* (Bl 40), and *Cheng Fu* (Bl 36).

2. Fiber-severing as instructed for hemorrhoids above.

Case history: A female, aged 46, complained of anal fissures and constipation with bleeding and pain on evacuation. She was treated by needling *Tian Shu* (St 25) to soften her stools and moxaing the local points. Five treatments and the patient recovered.

4
Sitting Wind (Perianal Eczema)

This disease is characterized by such an unbearable itching around the anus that the patient cannot enjoy sitting quiet for a moment, being unable to refrain from scratching frequently. Thus this disease acquires its name of sitting wind.

Disease causes, disease mechanisms

This disease is a product of wind, damp, and heat evils depressed in the skin surrounding the anus. These evils may be brewed by enduring dysentery or diarrhea, negligence of hygiene, or inhibited sweating due to various factors, for instance, overly tight pants.

Treatment principles: Clear heat and disinhibit dampness, dispel wind and stop itching

Formula: *Chang Qiang* (GV 1), *Hui Yang* (Bl 35), and *Bai Huan Shu* (Bl 30)

Treatment method: Prick around *Chang Qiang* (GV 1) to let out a bit of blood. Puncture the other two points to a shallow depth with a filiform needle.

Other choices:

1. Moxa the local points.

2. Steam and wash the affected area with hot salt water 1 time each day.

Book Seven: Tumors

What are called tumors and carcinomas in modern Western medicine are, in effect, a large number of different diseases in Chinese medicine. For example, conglomerations and concretions, locking anus hemorrhoid, mammary rock, esophageal constriction, and silkworm lip are all Chinese diseases covered by the modern medical concept of tumors and cancers.

Disease causes, disease mechanisms

Chinese medicine lays great store in the emotional factors or the seven affects as disease causes of tumors. However, external evils are also included as important pathogens.

Treatment based on pattern discrimination

Based on the above conception, tumors and carcinomas are divided into the following patterns:

1. Qi depression & stagnation pattern: Depression, worry, and anxiety may produce binding, causing the qi to counterflow in the liver and spleen and further block the channels and network vessels. Then this binding develops into something with a kernel. If the tumor feels hard, it is usually ascribed to qi depression. If the tumor is a nodulation with diffuse swelling, it often falls within the category of qi stagnation. In addition, in most cases, qi depression and stagnation are accompanied by chest and rib-side distention or abdominal glomus and distention.

Treatment principles: To treat this pattern, coursing the liver and rectifying the qi should take precedence over opening depression and scattering nodulation.

2. Blood stasis pattern: If the swollen mass is hard and the overlying skin is purplish or green-blue, or if red network-like veins are visible on the skin, this suggests a blood stasis pattern.

Treatment principles: To treat this pattern, one should quicken the blood and transform stasis through coursing the liver and rectifying the qi.

3. Congested phlegm pattern: Spleen vacuity makes it impossible for the spleen to transform and convey dampness. Therefore, dampness may gather and be boiled down by heat into phlegm.

This then will pour down into the spaces between the skin and flesh. This pattern, therefore, describes a cyst embracing a mass under the skin but over the muscular membrane.

Treatment principles: To treat this pattern, the practitioner should give priority to dispersing phlegm, softening the hard, and scattering nodulation through coursing the liver and rectifying the qi.

4. Gathered dampness pattern: This pattern describes a fluid-filled mass, ascites, or erosive exudation.

Treatment principles: To treat this pattern, priority should be given to dispersing swelling and transforming water through fortifying the spleen and boosting kidney yang.

5. Fire toxins pattern: This describes a hard mass with intense pain or festering with foul pus.

Treatment principles: This pattern can be successfully treated through enriching yin blood, boosting kidney water, and downbearing heart fire.

Dampness usually exhibits chest oppression and slimy tongue fur. Fire toxins gives rise to intense pain and tinges the skin a bright red color. Coughing of phlegm reveals gathered phlegm. These manifestations help diagnosis.

1
Goiter

In Chinese medicine, goiter is divided into qi goiter (simple diffuse thyroid adenoma), flesh goiter (thyroid adenoma), sinew goiter (angioma), and stone goiter (thyroid carcinoma). Here the discussion is limited to qi and flesh goiters.

Disease causes, disease mechanisms

As a disease, goiter appeared in the literature centuries earlier than *The Inner Classic*, and many scholars have since contributed to the lore about goiter in respect of its causes, treatment methods, etc. First of all, emotional disturbances are viewed as an important cause. Anxiety, worry, depression, and anger may give rise to liver depression. As a result, impairment of the spleen's movement and transformation arises. Then the qi becomes stagnant and phlegm accumulates. Stagnant qi and accumulated phlegm bind together so as to produce qi goiter.

Secondly, water and earth, a common Chinese construction implying food and weather in a given district, may cause this disease. *A Concise Book* says:

> In the central states, people contract goiter as a result of indignation producing binding. The goiter dangles with no core. In Changan (present day Xian) and Xiangyang, the natives drink sandy water and consequently are subject to growth of goiter with a kernel. The goiter is pendulous with no root, suspended within the skin. In these areas, the women who suffer from it have kidney qi repletion. Sand, being replete (meaning solid/hard) by nature, agrees with the kidneys, and hence makes the kidneys replete. As a result the disease goiter is produced.

Third, it was in the Ming dynasty that scholars began to include kidney vacuity as a cause of this disease. *Entering the Gate* says, "When the kidney qi sustains depletion and detriment, evils may take advantage of the vacuous channels during menstruation or delivery" to cause goiter.

To treat goiter, the modalities advanced by past outstanding medical figures included surgical operation, acumoxatherapy, etc. It is interesting to find that, among the other treatment alternatives, food containing iodine was suggested as an effective medicinal 2,000 years ago. The *Shen Nong Ben Cao Jing (The Divine Husbandman's Materia Medica Classic)*, which came out in the Han dynasty, prescribed marine algae to treat goiter.

Qi Goiter

1. Liver depression & damp phlegm pattern: Qi stagnation is manifest by exacerbation of the condition with emotional disturbance, menstrual flow, and pregnancy as well as by distention of the breasts and rib-side pain. Phlegm dampness may give rise to chest oppression, heart palpitations, weak limbs, and torpid intake. If there is the complication of spleen yang vacuity, there will be abdominal fullness, diarrhea, cold limbs, and glomus in the stomach duct.

Treatment principles: Course the liver and rectify the qi, transform phlegm and eliminate dampness

Formula: *He Gu* (LI 4), *Tian Tu* (CV 22), *Qu Chi* (LI 11), *Feng Chi* (GB 20), *Kun Lun* (Bl 60), local *a shi* points, and the *Hua Tuo Jia Ji* points from the 3rd to 5th cervical vertebra

Modifications: In case of qi stagnation, add *Nei Guan* (Per 6), *Zhong Zhu* (TB 3), *Yang Ling Quan* (GB 34), and *Wai Guan* (TB 5). In case of phlegm dampness, add *Zu San Li* (St 36), *Yin Ling Quan* (Sp 9), *Ren Ying* (St 9), and *Zhong Wan* (CV 12). In case of heart palpitations, add *Shen Men* (Ht 7) and *Tong Li* (Ht 5).

Treatment method: One often used *a shi* point is located a bit medial to *Shui Tu* (St 10). Insert a needle at this point towards the center of the goiter, and then, after withdrawing the needle a little, thrust it deep at different angles. This technique is called cock claw needling. Sometimes this point can be replaced by 3-5 cervical paravertebral points. In addition, 1-2 points around the periphery of the goiter can be chosen. When puncturing *He Gu* (LI 4), strong stimulation is allowed. Other points are needled in the conventional way.

Explanation of the formula: The local points, including *Tian Tu* (CV 22) and *Ren Ying* (St 9), are expected to course and free the flow of the local channel qi to directly disperse swelling and scatter nodulation. *Zu San Li* (St 36), *Zhong Wan* (CV 12), and *Yin Ling Quan* (Sp 9) are used to fortify the spleen to move dampness and transform phlegm. *Shen Men* (Ht 7) and *Tong Li* (Ht 5) calm the spirit. *Nei Guan* (Per 6), *Wai Guan* (TB 5), *Yang Ling Quan* (GB 34), and *Zhong Zhu* (TB 3) are able to course the liver and rectify the qi as well as disinhibit the triple burner. *He Gu* (LI 4) and *Qu Chi* (LI 11) are used to harmonize and balance the qi and blood because the *yang ming* channel is abundant in both qi and blood.

2. Yin vacuity & hyperactive fire pattern: This pattern is characterized by irascibility or emotional depression, insomnia, profuse sweating, a red facial complexion, a bitter taste in the mouth, vexation, emaciation despite large food intake, and a red tongue body with yellow fur.

Treatment principles: Enrich yin, clear fire, and calm the spirit

Formula: *Nei Guan* (Per 6), *Zu San Li* (St 36), *He Gu* (LI 4), and the *a shi* points

Modifications: In case of yin vacuity and effulgent fire, add *Jian Shi* (Per 5), *Shen Men* (Ht 7), *San Yin Jiao* (Sp 6), *Tai Chong* (Liv 3), *Tai Xi* (Ki 3), and *Fu Liu* (Ki 7). In case of qi vacuity in addition to yin vacuity, add *Guan Yuan* (CV 4), *Zhao Hai* (Ki 6), *San Yin Jiao* (Sp 6), and *Fu Liu* (Ki 7).

Treatment method: Needle using supplementing technique. The *a shi* points often used in practice are four points located 0.5 *cun* above and below *Ren Ying* (St 9).

Flesh Goiter

This type of goiter feels hard and is often oval-shaped with a smooth surface.

Treatment principles: Course the liver and resolve depression, rectify the qi and transform phlegm, soften the hard and scatter nodulation

Formula: *Shui Tu* (St 10), *Tian Tu* (CV 22), *Tian Ding* (LI 17), and the *a shi* points

Treatment method: Needle as instructed above.

Other choices:

1. Needle *Tian Ding* (LI 17), *Fu Tu* (LI 18), *Qi She* (St 11), *Tai Chong* (Liv 3), *Nei Guan* (Per 6), *San Li* (St 36), *Yin Ling Quan* (Sp 9), and the *a shi* point which is the center of the goiter. Puncture the local *a shi* point with a red-hot needle. Needle the other points using draining technique.

2. Moxa 3-5 points in 1 treatment chosen from *Tian Tu* (CV 22), *Tong Tian* (Bl 7), *Yun Men* (Lu 2), *Bi Nao* (LI 14), *Qu Chi* (LI 11), *Zhong Feng* (Liv 14), *Shan Zhong* (CV 17), *Feng Chi* (GB 20), *Da Zhui* (GV 14), *Qi She* (St 11), *Tian Fu* (Lu 3), and *Chong Yang* (St 42).

3. Tap the local *a shi* points with a cutaneous needle until they bleed slightly 1 time each day.

Reference: In a study of qi goiter and acupuncture, if the goiter was small and grew on one side of the neck, then *Shui Tu* (St 10) on the affected side was punctured. The needle was inserted 2/3 into the goiter. Then cock claw needling was performed. If the goiter was large, then one needle was inserted at *Shui Tu* and another needle was inserted on either side of *Shui Tu*. If the goiter occupied both sides of the neck, then *Shui Tu* was punctured bilaterally, and then another needle was inserted 5 *fen* lateral to the point on either side. *He Gu* (LI 4) or *Lie Que* (Lu 7) might be needled as an auxiliary point. Ninety-five cases of simple thyroid adenoma were treated by this technique. Of these, 17 recovered; 15 showed noticeable improvement; 50 became better; and 13 reported no response. The total effectiveness rate was 87%. Jin Shu-bai *et al: Zhong Guo Zhen Jiu (Chin. Acu. & Mox.)* 1982; (1):14.

2
Tofu-dregs Tumor (Sebaceous Cyst)

Disease causes, disease mechanisms

The Orthodox Gathering says:

> Whenever fluids and foam stagnate in the interstices, they will gather, refusing to disperse. Then they will gradually develop into this species of tumor... It often recurs (after having been cured), for there is a cyst.

Treatment principles: Warm to free the flow of the qi and blood, quicken the network vessels and dissipate stasis

Treatment choices:

1. Puncture the center of the tumor with a red-hot needle.

2. Moxa the tumor directly or over ginger or garlic.

Case history: A male, aged 29, had a mass the size of a peach kernel near *Da Zhui* (GV 14). This caused no pain but did cause a sensation of heaviness. After routine sterilization, a red-hot needle was inserted into the center of the mass and then quantities of semiliquid substances were pressed out from the needle hole. Finally, the cyst was removed with a hemostat after being cleaned. Five days later, the wound healed. No infection and no recurrence was found on follow-up.

Reference: There is a report of 50 cases of sebaceous cyst on the face and neck treated by fire-needling. Forty-six cases were healed. Luan Shu-fen: *Zhong Guo Zhen Jiu (Chin. Acu. & Mox.)* 1995; 15 (6):19.

3
Mammary Node (Mammary Fibroadenoma) (1)

Mammary node is also called breast aggregation. It is divided in modern Western medicine into two different species, breast fibroadenoma and cystic hyperplasia.

Disease causes, disease mechanisms

In the *Wai Ke Shu Yao (The Pivotal Essentials of External Medicine)* published in 1571 CE, the author, Xue Ji, gave a good analysis of the disease, saying:

> Breast aggregation is a hard node in the breast. At the beginning, it is the size of a coin and grows little by little to the size of a peach or even an egg, with the overlying skin normal in color. When subjected to cold, it gives pain. It is produced by a cold form (*i.e.*, body) and limbs in conspiracy with qi depression and phlegm rheum which flow into the stomach network vessels, gathering, accumulating, and not dispersing. With effulgent qi and at young ages, it may last for one or two years... and then disperse. Those who are elderly with debilitated qi and who suffer from it for years are incurable. It is necessary (for them) to be abstemious of food and drink and (to avoid) vexation and anger to prevent transmutation into mammary rock (*i.e.*, breast cancer).

Treatment based on pattern discrimination

As far as breast fibroadenoma is concerned, clinically there are three different patterns:

1. Liver depression & phlegm congelation pattern: Emotional depression damages the liver, causing qi to be depressed and phlegm to gather. Depressed qi and accumulated phlegm settle in the stomach network vessels in the breast. Worry and anxiety may damage the spleen, which is the viscus of damp earth and which has an interior-exterior relationship with the stomach. When the spleen and stomach are not in harmony, they fail to transform and convey water dampness. When dampness accumulates, it develops into phlegm, blocking the network vessels. When the qi and blood are inhibited, binding or nodulation appears. The nipple is ascribed to the liver channel, while the breast to the stomach channel. In sum, therefore, these two channels should be held responsible for this disease.

This pattern is distinguished by such signs and symptoms as vexation, irascibility, chest oppression, shortness of breath, insomnia, profuse dreaming, a red tongue, and a rapid, bowstring or slippery, bowstring pulse.

Treatment principles: Course the liver and rectify the qi, transform phlegm and scatter nodulation

Formula: *Wu Yi* (St 15), *Shan Zhong* (CV 17), *Xing Jian* (Liv 2), *Ying Chuang* (St 16), *Feng Long* (St 40), *Pi Shu* (Bl 20), *Zhong Wan* (CV 12), and *a shi* points

Treatment method: Needle using draining technique except for the *a shi* points. Prick and then perform cupping over 3-5 local *a shi* points.

Explanation of the formula: Since the breasts are on the route of the foot *yang ming*, distant and local points on the *yang ming* are able to move the channel qi to resolve congestion and stagnation. In addition, the distant point, *Feng Long* (St 40), is markedly specific for phlegm. *Xing Jian* (Liv 2) is the spring point of the liver channel and hence is able to course the liver and resolve depression as well as to clear fire from the liver. When combined with it, *Pi Shu* (Bl 20) and *Zhong Wan* (CV 12)'s action on the spleen is strengthened. When the spleen is fortified, it is able to transform phlegm and the central qi is freed. Once the central qi enjoys free circulation, the blood will move and the network vessels will be unblocked. As a result of the combined work of these points, nodulations are scattered and swelling dispersed.

2. Penetrating & controlling vessel disharmony pattern: The penetrating vessel is the sea of blood, while the controlling vessel governs the uterus. If a woman suffers long from menstrual troubles, the penetrating and controlling vessels will be affected. As a result, qi and blood interfere with one another, forming a binding or nodulation.

This pattern is established if there are such complications as menstrual irregularity, fatigue, and weak and aching low back and knees.

Treatment principles: Balance the penetrating and controlling vessels, disperse accumulation and scatter nodulation

Formula: *Guan Yuan* (CV 4), *Shui Quan* (Ki 5), *Li Gou* (Liv 5), *Shen Shu* (Bl 23), *Ru Gen* (St 18), *Wei Bao* (located 5 *fen* medial to *Wu Chu* [Bl 5]), and *a shi* points

Treatment method: Needle using draining technique at *Ru Gen* (St 18) and supplementation at the other points except the *a shi* points. The *a shi* points are the points surrounding the swelling, 2-4 in number.

Explanation of the formula: *Guan Yuan* (CV 4) is a point on the controlling vessel, but it connects with the foot *shao yin* and penetrating vessel. Therefore, it is vital for boosting the source qi and balancing the penetrating and controlling vessels. *Shui Quan* (Ki 5), the cleft point of the foot *shao yin*, and *Li Gou* (Liv 5), the connecting point of the foot *jue yin*, act synergistically in supplementing the liver and kidneys and securing the penetrating and controlling vessels.

3. Qi & blood vacuity pattern: This pattern is characterized by pain in the breasts which is worse with taxation and fatigue. There may be the complications of torpid intake, dizziness arising on movement, spontaneous sweating, heart palpitations, drowsiness, a lusterless facial complexion, and emaciation. The pulse is deep and fine.

Treatment principles: Supplement the qi and nourish blood, support the righteous and scatter nodulations

Formula: *Qi Hai* (CV 6), *Guan Yuan* (CV 4), *San Li* (St 36), *Pi Shu* (Bl 20), *Wei Shu* (Bl 21), *Shen Shu* (Bl 23), *Shan Zhong* (CV 17), *Nei Guan* (Per 6), and local *a shi* points

Treatment method: Needle using supplementing technique except for the *a shi* points. The *a shi* points, which are the center of each of the nodes, are punctured with mugwort burned on the heads of the needles during retention.

Explanation of the formula: *Qi Hai* (Sea of Qi, CV 6), as its name suggests, is particularly good at rectifying and boosting the qi, and its action is enhanced when it is used in combination with *Guan Yuan* (CV 4). These two points also balance the penetrating and controlling vessels. Acting synergistically with these two, *Shen Shu* (Bl 23) is able to supplement the former heaven or prenatal qi, while *Pi Shu* (Bl 20) and *Wei Shu* (Bl 21) are intended to supplement the postnatal or central qi. *Shan Zhong* (CV 17) is the sea of qi and can promote circulation of qi in the chest. When the qi is greatly supplemented and boosted, the blood will move and binding or nodulations will be dispersed.

Other choices:

1. Needle the node, *San Li* (St 36), and *Tai Chong* (Liv 3) or *Qi Men* (Liv 14). Add *Feng Long* (St 40) for the liver depression pattern. Add *San Yin Jiao* (Sp 6) and *Tai Xi* (Ki 3) for penetrating and controlling disharmony pattern.

2. Moxa the node directly or over ginger 1 time each day.

3. Press or puncture the auricular points Endocrine (MA-IC3), Liver (MA-SC5), Kidney (MA), and Mammary Gland.

Case history: A female, aged 32, came for treatment in April 1985. She complained of a mass as large as an egg in her left breast. The node felt smooth, a little painful, and distended. The case had been diagnosed as breast fibroadenoma, and surgery had been recommended. Because the patient was afraid of the operation, she chose acumoxatherapy. This case was determined as liver depression and phlegm congelation pattern. The treatment consisted of rounding-up puncturing, meaning that several, typically 4, needles were inserted around the edges of the node obliquely downward toward the center of the node. To soothe the liver, *Tai Chong* (Liv 3) was also punctured. The treatment was given 1 time every other day. Ten sessions dispersed the node completely.

Reference: There is a report on the treatment of breast fibroadenoma with the DM701-IIA electroacuanesthetizer. The points needled were *Wu Yi* (St 15), *Shan Zhong* (CV 17), and *He Gu* (LI 4). *Tai Chong* (Liv 3) was added in case of effulgent liver fire. *Shen Shu* (Bl 23) and *Tai Xi* (Ki 3) were added in case of liver-kidney yin vacuity and/or after menstruation. *San Li* (St 36) and *Pi Shu* (Bl 20) were added in case of insufficiency of qi and blood. *San Yin Jiao* (Sp 6) was added in case of menstrual irregularity and/or before menstruation. The anesthetizer was adjusted to the maximum power that the patient could bear. Treatment was performed 6-8, 13-15, or 22-27 days after menstruation. A comparison with other modalities was made, and the results of this method were most satisfactory. Liu Li-jun: *Zhong Guo Zhen Jiu (Chin. Acu. & Mox.)* 1996; 16(4):7.

4
Mammary Node (Fibrocystic Breast Condition) (2)

Disease causes, disease mechanisms

From the point of view of Chinese medicine, the disease causes of this condition are the same as for fibroadenoma.

Treatment based on pattern discrimination

Fibrocystic breast condition is categorized as the following patterns:

1. Liver depression & qi stagnation pattern: This is probably the most common pattern of this condition seen in clinical practice. It is characterized by melancholy, disinclination to speak, diminished qi, and irritability. The tongue is red with white fur, and the pulse is bowstring.

2. Penetrating & controlling vessel disharmony pattern: There is menstrual irregularity. The mass increases in size and the pain gets worse towards menstruation. The tongue is possibly normal in color with white fur, and the pulse is bowstring and fine.

3. Qi stagnation & blood stasis pattern: The mass becomes more painful with the beginning or ending of the menstrual flow and with emotional disturbances like anger and anxiety. There may be chest and rib-side pain, distention, and oppression. The tongue is red with white fur and with possible static spots or macules on the tongue. The pulse is bowstring and fine.

4. Blood stasis & toxins gathering pattern: There is a painful, swollen mass which enlarges comparatively rapidly. The pain gets worse towards the menstrual flow and may be accompanied by vexation and agitation, insomnia, and profuse dreaming. The pain also gets worse with emotional disturbance.

5. Qi & blood vacuity pattern: This pattern is often seen in enduring cases which have been repeatedly administered cool and cold medicinals. The patient, who usually has a white facial complexion, is short of breath, listless, and easily fatigued. Their appetite is poor and there is possible slight swelling in the lower legs.

6. Spleen & kidney vacuity pattern: The patient suffers from aversion to cold with constantly chilled limbs. There is also foamy sputum, torpid intake, 2-3 bowel movements per day with loose stools or untransformed grains (in the stool), reduced sexual desire, difficult conception, liability to miscarriage, weakness, and fatigue. The tongue is pale with white fur, and the pulse is deep, fine, and weak.

Treatment principles: Soften the hard and scatter nodulation, course the network vessels of the breast and resolve depression

Formula: *Shan Zhong* (CV 17), *Ru Gen* (St 18), and *Wu Yi* (St 15)

Modifications: For pattern #1, add *Qi Men* (Liv14) and *Tai Chong* (Liv 3) using draining technique. For pattern #2, add *Guan Yuan* (CV 4) and *Shen Shu* (Bl 23) using even manipulation, *i.e.*, neither supplementation nor drainage. For pattern #3, add *Nei Guan* (Per 6), *Ge Shu* (Bl 17), and *Tai Chong* (Liv 3) using draining technique. For pattern #4, add *San Yin Jiao* (Sp 6) and *Wei Zhong* (Bl 40), pricking the latter. For pattern #5, add *San Li* (St 36), *San Yin Jiao* (Sp 6), and *Guan Yuan* (CV 4), needling and then moxaing. For pattern #6, add *Guan Yuan* (CV 4) and *Ming Men* (GV 4), moxaing.

Other choice: 1. Orally administer formulas based on *Xiao Yao San* (Rambling Powder) which is composed of: Radix Bupleuri (*Chai Hu*), Radix Angelicae Sinensis (*Dang Gui*), Radix Albus Paeoniae Lactiflorae (*Bai Shao*), Rhizoma Atractylodis Macrocephalae (*Bai Zhu*), Sclerotium Poriae Cocos (*Fu Ling*), Herba Menthae Haplocalycis (*Bo He*), and Radix Glycyrrhizae (*Gan Cao*). The formula should be varied in accordance with particular patterns. To course the liver and resolve depression, the medicinals to be selected include: Radix Bupleuri (*Chai Hu*), Pericarpium Citri Reticulatae Viride (*Qing Pi*), Rhizoma Cyperi Rotundi (*Xiang Fu*), Radix Albus Peoniae Lactiflorae (*Bai Shao*), Fructus Meliae Toosendan (*Chuan Lian Zi*), and Radix Platycodi Grandiflori (*Jie Geng*). To transform phlegm and soften the hard, the medicinals often prescribed include: Thallus Algae (*Kun Bu*), Herba Sargassii (*Hai Zao*), Concha Ostreae (*Mu Li*), Bulbus Fritillariae (*Bei Mu*), Spica Prunellae Vulgaris (*Xia Ku Cao*), Semen Sinapis Albae (*Bai Jie Zi*), and Bulbus Shancigu (*Shan Ci Gu*). To quicken the blood and transform stasis, the choices often used are: Radix Rubrus Paeoniae Lactiflorae (*Chi Shao*), Rhizoma Curcumae Zedoariae (*E Zhu*), Tuber Curcumae (*Yu Jin*), Semen Vaccariae Segetalis (*Wang Bu Liu Xing*), etc. To boost the qi, nourish the blood, and supplement the liver and kidneys, one may choose from: Radix Polygoni Multiflori (*He Shou Wu*), Radix Glycyrrhizae (*Gan Cao*), Radix Astragali Membranacei (*Huang Qi*), Cortex Cinnamomi Cassiae (*Rou Gui*), and Herba Epimedii (*Yin Yang Huo*).

Note: For this condition, Chinese practitioners usually prefer a combination of acumoxatherapy and medication, since medication alone often fails to achieve a permanent effect. In addition, modern Chinese physicians often add some yang-invigorating agents like Herba Epimedii (*Xian*

Ling Pi), Semen Cuscutae (*Tu Si Zi*), Rhizoma Curculiginis Orchioidis (*Xian Mao*), and Cortex Eucommiae Ulmoidis (*Du Zhong*).

Reference: There is a report of 500 cases of mammary hyperplasia treated by acupuncture. The points needled included *Wu Yi* (St 15), *Shan Zhong* (CV 17), *He Gu* (LI 4), *Tian Zong* (SI 11), *Jian Jing* (GB 21), and *Gan Shu* (Bl 18). Supplementation or drainage was performed depending on vacuity and repletion. Of these cases, 227 were cured. The total effectiveness rate was 95%. Guo Cheng-jie: *Zhong Guo Zhen Jiu (Chin. Acu. & Mox.)* 1986; (4):2.

Book Eight: Postoperative & Miscellaneous Troubles

In modern times, Chinese acupuncturists have been faced with the new problem of postoperative complaints. This proves that acupuncture and moxibustion can add effective alternatives to modern Western medicine in combatting these disorders and promoting rehabilitation. Surgery unavoidably damages the righteous qi and leaves behind inhibition of the qi and blood. This results in postoperative pain, and, as the saying goes:

> If there is lack of free flow, there is pain.
> If there is pain, there is lack of free flow.

Surgery may also result in postoperative urinary block because inhibited qi is unable to command the water passageways. Because the central qi is damaged, nausea, retching and vomiting, abdominal distention, and constipation may also all appear postoperatively. This section also includes some nonsurgical wounds or sores which are of a similar nature as postoperative complaints.

1
Helping Heal the Cut

Because surgical operation damages the righteous qi, healing of the incision may be retarded, and, in many cases, there are the complications of pain, festering, and numbness. This is most often seen in cases of weak physique.

Treatment choices: To treat a cut refusing to close, one may first apply some disinfectant and then moxa the local points. For a mild case, a couple of such treatments may heal the wound. If the case has lasted for a long time, one may moxa and then apply some herbal powder. If there are rotten tissues, one may prescribe *Qu Fu San* (Dispel Rot Powder). This is composed of: Resina Olibani (*Ru Xiang*), Resina Myrrhae (*Mo Yao*), Cinnabar (*Zhu Sha*), Calomelas (*Qing Fen*), and Serpent's Bezoar (*i.e.*, Pisiform Clay Iron Ore, *She Han Shi*). If there is not yet rotten flesh, one may apply powdered Cortex Radicis Lycii (*Di Gu Pi*) or Cortex Phellodendri (*Huang*

Bai) or *Sheng Ji San* (Generate Muscle [*i.e.*, Flesh] Powder). This is composed of: Radix Auklandiae Lappae (*Mu Xiang*), Semen Arecae Catechu (*Bing Lang*), and Rhizoma Coptidis Chinensis (*Huang Lian*).

Case histories:

A 16 year old male was wounded in his right lateral malleolus in a traffic accident. The wound refused to heal for over 20 days and developed an ulcer in the affected area with a diameter of 3cm along with some rotten flesh. The treatment principles were to simply warm and free the flow of the qi and blood in order to generate muscle (*i.e.*, flesh). The local points and the lesion proper were moxaed, and *Sheng Ji San* was applied. Treatment was given 1 time every other day, and 7 sessions healed the wound.

A 4 year old male suffered from a suppurative wound from which the sutures had yet to be removed. After debridement, moxibustion was carried out and then *Qu Fu San* was applied. Treatment was given 1 time every other day. Ten days of treatment effected a cure.

2
Postoperative Nausea, Retching & Vomiting

Following digestive system surgery, stubborn retching and vomiting may appear.

Treatment principles: Harmonize the stomach and downbear counterflow, fortify the spleen and rectify the qi

Formula: *Nei Guan* (Per 6), *Zhong Wan* (CV 12), *San Li* (St 36), *Tian Shu* (St 25), *Liang Men* (St 21), and *Gong Sun* (Sp 4)

Treatment method: Needle using draining technique. If there is central qi vacuity, use supplementation.

Explanation of the formula: *Nei Guan* (Per 6) is a proven point which is very good at suppressing nausea and retching and vomiting. *Zhong Wan* (CV 12) strongly rectifies the qi of the middle burner and fortifies the spleen and stomach since it is both the alarm point of the stomach and a meeting point of the hand *tai yang*, hand *shao yang*, foot *yang ming*, and controlling vessel. Combined with it, *San Li* (St 36) and *Gong Sun* (Sp 4) are strengthened in their action of harmonizing the spleen and stomach and downbearing counterflow. *Tian Shu* (St 25), the alarm point of the large intestine, works as a pivot of the qi mechanism of the stomach and intestines. As such, it is good at normalizing the middle burner and downbearing counterflowing qi. *Liang Men* (St 21) is the gate for the entrance and exit of the stomach qi. Therefore, it fortifies the spleen, rectifies the central qi, and harmonizes the stomach.

Case history: A female, aged 52, had undergone surgery for lung cancer 20 days previously. The patient suffered from inability to take in food, retching and vomiting, and acid regurgitation. Western medicines and Chinese medicinals had proven ineffective. The clinical findings of a deep, weak pulse, a pale facial complexion, a pink tongue body with white, slimy fur, fatigued expression, and disinclination to speak supported the diagnosis of spleen vacuity with damp obstruction. This then underlay the treatment principles of supporting the righteous and fortifying the spleen, transforming dampness and dispelling evils. The treatment consisted of a combination of needling and moxibustion. Thus *Nei Guan* (Per 6) and *Zhong Wan* (CV 12) were needled, while *Guan Yuan* (CV 4), *San Li* (St 36), and *San Yin Jiao* (Sp 6) were moxaed. Treatment was given 1 time each day, and 5 sessions effected basic relief of the troubles. Then, moxibustion of *Guan Yuan* and *San Li* was continued in order to promote general rehabilitation.

3
Postoperative Abdominal Distention & Constipation

Disease causes, disease mechanisms

Surgery, and particularly that for abdominal problems, often damages the yang qi of the bowels so that the clear yang is not upborne, while the turbid yin is not downborne. Thus the bowel qi is blocked and held up in the intestines. Nausea, inability to take in food, and shortness of breath may also arise besides abdominal distention and constipaton.

Treatment principles: Boost the qi and eliminate fullness

Formula: *San Li* (St 36), *Zhong Wan* (CV 12), *Tian Shu* (St 25), and *Shen Que* (CV 8)

Treatment method: Needle, moxa, or combine needling and moxibustion, choosing from the above points and using supplementation or drainage depending upon vacuity or repletion, except for the last point on which needling is not allowed.

Other choices:

1. Press while rubbing the umbilicus clockwise for 2 minutes.

2. Needle *San Li* (St 36) and *Nei Ting* (St 44) with strong stimulation and then moxa them.

Case history: A male, aged 32 suffered from severe abdominal distention accompanied by nausea, chest oppression, no desire for food, and rib-side pain following surgery for appendicitis. The patient had thick, slimy tongue fur and a rapid, bowstring pulse. *San Li* (St 36) was needled bilaterally with draining hand technique. The instant the needle sensation was obtained, thunderous flatulence was induced and abdominal distention was removed.

Note: I have treated more than 10 similar cases by needling *San Li* (St 36). All these cases got relief within 2 hours after needling. However, a few had a relapse. In that case, 2-3 more treatments were needed.

4
Hiccough

Hiccough may be an independent disorder or merely a complication of some other disease. Sometimes it is not only annoying but dangerous. It has been a topic in many old medical classics since *The Inner Classic*. Although this disorder is placed under the post-operative category in this particular book, it is more often seen outside this situation and its causes and mechanisms are manifold.

Disease causes, disease mechanisms

If surgical operation damages stomach yin and the stomach network vessels, then the stomach qi will be plunged into disorder. As a result, it stops descending but counterflows upwards. With counterflow of stomach qi, the diaphragm is stirred up, giving rise to hiccough. Eating too much cold or acrid food or medicinals may also lead to stomach qi counterflow. As the stomach qi keeps on going up without descending, the diaphragm qi will be inhibited. As a result, diaphragm striking (*da ge*), the literal translation of the Chinese name for this disorder, occurs. Hiccough may also be impugned to phlegm. Indignation, anger, and depression may obstruct the qi and hence the flow of fluids may become inhibited. Accumulated fluids transform into phlegm. Since emotional disturbances may cause liver depression and qi counterflow, this counterflow drafts this phlegm upward, striking the diaphragm. And finally, depletion of the righteous qi, which often occurs in enduring disease or as the result of abusing ejection and precipitation, may cause stomach qi disharmony. This may even involve the kidneys which lose their functions of qi-containing and securing. In either case, the diaphragm qi will be stirred.

Treatment based on pattern discrimination

In the *Zheng Zhi Hui Bu (Collected Supplements to [the Theory of] Patterns & Treatment)* by Li Yong-cui published in 1687 CE, there is a passage devoted to the identification of the different patterns of hiccough. It says:

> Fire hiccough is a loud, recurrent hiccough accompanied by intense thirst, difficult urination, and a rapid, forceful pulse. Cold hiccough is characterized by relief in the morning and exacerbation in the evening. It is continual and is accompanied by chilled hands and feet and a slow, weak pulse. Phlegm hiccough is hiccough with phlegm rales accompanied by inhibited breathing and a slippery yet weak

pulse. Vacuity hiccough is characterized by gasping for breath despite loud hiccoughing and a vacuous, weak pulse. Stasis hiccough is characterized by pricking pain in the chest, hiccoughing on drinking water, and a scallion-stalk, deep, choppy pulse.

Treatment principles: Harmonize the stomach and downbear counterflow

Formula: a) *San Li* (St 36), *Zhong Wan* (CV 12), and *Nei Guan* (Per 6); b) *Tian Tu* (CV 22) and *Shan Zhong* (CV 17); c) *Ge Shu* (Bl 17) and *Ju Que* (CV 14)

Treatment method: Needle one or two points from each group in one treatment. Puncture *San Li* (St 36) and *Nei Guan* (Per 6) using lifting and thrusting hand technique to provoke strong stimulation. It is better yet to puncture *San Li* with a warm needle. At *Tian Tu* (CV 22), the needle is inserted subcutaneously parallel to the sternum.

Modifications: In case of liver qi overwhelming the stomach, add *Tai Chong* (Liv 3) and *Yang Ling Quan* (GB 34) to course the liver and rectify the qi. In case of lung qi refusing to descend, add *Tai Yuan* (Lu 9) and *Chi Ze* (Lu 5) to downbear the lung qi. In case of binding and stagnation of the intestines, add *Tian Shu* (St 25) and *Nei Ting* (St 44) to free the bowels and abduct stagnation. In case of kidneys unable to secure the qi, add *Tai Xi* (Ki 3), *Guan Yuan* (CV 4), and *Qi Hai* (CV 6) to supplement the kidneys.

Explanation of the formula: *San Li* (St 36) is the sea point of the foot *yang ming*. *Zhong Wan* (CV 12) is the alarm point of the stomach, the meeting point of the bowels, and is also a meeting point of the hand *tai yin*, hand *shao yang*, foot *yang ming*, and controlling vessel. *Nei Guan* (Per 6) is the network point of the hand *jue yin* and a meeting point of the eight vessels connecting with the yin linking vessel. Working together, these three points harmonize the stomach and downbear counterflow. *Tian Tu* (CV 22) is a meeting point of the yin linking and controlling vessels. *Shan Zhong* (CV 17) is the meeting point of the qi and a meeting point of the foot *tai yin*, foot *shao yin*, hand *tai yang*, hand *shao yang*, and controlling vessel. These two points combined together are able to loosen the chest and disinhibit the diaphragm qi, diffuse the lungs and downbear counterflow. *Ge Shu* (Bl 17) is the back transporting point of the diaphragm and the meeting point of blood, while *Ju Que* (CV 14) is the alarm point of the heart. The combination of these two points can rectify the qi and harmonize the blood, dispel phlegm and open the diaphragm.

Other choices:

1. Moxa *Shan Zhong* (CV 17), *Zhong Wan* (CV 12), and *Guan Yuan* (CV 4) with cones or a moxa roll for 20-30 minutes per treatment.

2. Electroacupuncture *Zhong Wan* (CV 12), *Ge Shu* (Bl 17), *Nei Guan* (Per 6), and *San Li* (St 36).

3. Perform cupping over *Ge Shu* (Bl 17), *Ge Guan* (Bl 46), and *Zhong Wan* (CV 12).

4. Press *Zan Zhu* (Bl 2) bilaterally with gradually increasing force for 3-5 minutes or press *Tian Zong* (SI 11), *Yi Feng* (TB 17), or the eyeballs till a sore and distended sensation appears.

5. Startling the patient may check hiccough if it is due to temporary emotional disturbance.

Case history: A male, aged 60, suffered from persistent hiccough following gastrectomy. Pressing *Zan Zhu* (Bl 2) with the edge of the thumb stopped the hiccoughing instantly.

Note: I have treated more than 10 cases with the same method and all were cured.

Reference: In his *Wai Ke Jing Yao (Pithy Essentials of External Medicine)*, Chen Zi-ming (1109-1170 CE) gives an account of his treatment of hiccough. A patient who had dysentery suffered from incessant hiccoughing which was recalcitrant to various prescriptions of medicinals. Then Chen moxaed *Qi Men* (Liv 14) with 3 cones and the hiccough was checked. Another patient suffered from incessant hiccoughing due to qi counterflow. Chen first needled *Shan Zhong* (CV 17) to open the path for qi and then *Qi Hai* (CV 6) to meet the qi coming from above. Then a cure was effected immediately. This method and the explanation of its curative effect implies that hiccough is caused by disruption of the qi.

5
Urinary Block (Urinary Retention)

Urinary block is seldom an independent disorder. (However,) it often exists as a complication of other diseases. In most cases, it is very dangerous. In the *Jing Yue Quan Shu (Jing-yue's Complete Book)*, the author, Zhang Jie-bin (1563-1640 CE), said:

> Inhibition of the water (passageways) is as good as urinary dribbling and complete block which is a most critical illness... In that event, it may threaten one's life.

Therefore, although urinary block is regarded as a branch disease, one should give priority to it in treatment.

Disease causes, disease mechanisms

The disease lies in the bladder, but it is due to failure of qi transformation for which the kidneys are responsible. This situation arises when the kidney qi sustains vacuity detriment and the fire of the life gate is debilitated. External injury, damage done by surgical operation, etc. may all damage the kidney qi and life gate fire. Therefore, this is an illness of root vacuity. Furthermore, its cause is often traced to lung metal because the lungs are the viscus that governs the water passageways through the qi. From another point of view, however, this is an illness of repletion. This is because, in such cases, damp heat inevitably pours down into the bladder. Thus this is a condition of root vacuity with branch repletion.

Treatment principles: Supplement the spleen and kidneys to facilitate qi transformation of water, clear damp heat to dissipate stasis and binding

Formula: *Zhong Ji* (CV 3), *Shui Dao* (St 28), *San Yin Jiao* (Sp 6), and *Gui Lai* (St 29)

Treatment method: Needle, electroacupuncture, or combine needling and moxibustion.

Explanation of the formula: Because *Zhong Ji* (CV 3) is the alarm point of the urinary bladder and a meeting point of the controlling vessel with the three foot yin channels, it is able to course the water passageways, free the bladder, and regulate the controlling vessel. *San Yin Jiao* (Sp 6) is the meeting point of the three foot yin channels and hence is good at harmonizing the qi and blood. It is chosen in order to act synergistically with *Zhong Ji*, since the combination of a distant and an adjacent point may connect the qi into a whole. *Shui Dao* (Waterway, St 28), as its name suggests, is a specific point for water problems able to open the water sluice.

Other choices:

1. Moxa *Shen Que* (CV 8) over salt.

2. Press and rub *Ji Men* (Sp 11) 200-500 times or press *Zhong Ji* (CV 3).

3. Puncture the auricular points Kidney (MA), Bladder (MA-SC8), Brain (Nao), and Sympathetic (MA-AH7).

4. Tap *Ci Liao* (Bl 32), *Pang Guang Shu* (Bl 28), and *San Jiao Shu* (Bl 22) with a cutaneous needle.

Case history: A male, aged 29, suffered from recalcitrant urinary retention following surgical operation for hemorrhoids. The patient had been catheterized many times but was still not able to void urine independently. He was given warm needling at *Zhong Ji* (CV 3) alone. One treatment cured the trouble.

Note: I have treated 23 similar cases. In most cases, I just needled *Zhong Ji* (CV 3) and *San Yin Jiao* (Sp 6) and achieved a cure in 1 treatment. In a few cases, 2 sessions were needed. I have also tried with success pressing *Zhong Ji* or *Guan Yuan* (CV 4). My experience fully attests to the miraculous effect of acupuncture on urinary retention.

6
External Kidney Welling Abscess (Acute Orchitis)

Welling abscess of the "external kidneys", *i.e.*, the testicles, falls within the category of prominent mounding (*shan*). This disease is usually characterized by sudden onset, pain, and a sagging sensation in the testicles often accompanied by fever, nausea, and headache. The pain may extend along the medial aspect of the thigh to the lower abdomen.

Disease causes, disease mechanisms

This disease is due to damp heat generated internally by overeating fatty, sweet, and rich flavors. This internally generated damp heat then pours downward along the liver channel, causing congestion and stagnation of the qi and blood, blocking the channels and network vessels. Such damage of the channels and network vessels with stasis and stagnation of the qi and blood may get worse by taxation and vacuity of the qi and blood. Thus evil heat becomes effulgent and putrefies the flesh. Hence external kidney welling abscess arises.

Treatment principles: Clear heat and resolve toxins, quicken the blood and disperse swelling

Formula: *Tai Chong* (Liv 3), *Xing Jian* (Liv 2), *Li Gou* (Liv 5), *Da Dun* (Liv 1), *Zhong Ji* (CV 3), and *San Yin Jiao* (Sp 6)

Treatment method: Needle using draining technique.

Explanation of the formula: The liver channel encircles the external genitals and hence is most closely related with troubles in the genitalia. Based on this understanding, pertinent points on the foot *jue yin* are selected to clear heat from the liver and resolve toxins. *San Yin Jiao* (Sp 6) is a meeting point of the three foot yin channels. As such, on one hand, it is able to fortify the spleen and transform dampness, and, on the other, it enriches kidney water. This is necessary because the testicles are, in practice, an extension of the kidneys.

Other choices:

1. Moxibustion: Ruling points: *Da Dun* (Liv 1), *Yong Quan* (Ki 1), *San Yin Jiao* (Sp 6), *Yang Chi* (TB 4), and triangular points. The triangular points, which are in fact two points, are measured

in the following way: Take the width of the mouth as one side of an equalateral triangle. Place the top angle of the triangle at the center of the navel. This angle will be bisected by the midline of the abdomen. Mark the points where the other two angles (of the base of the triangle) then fall. These are the so-called triangular points. Auxiliary points: *Tai Chong* (Liv 3), *Xing Jian* (Liv 2), *Shen Que* (CV 8), *Guan Yuan* (CV 4), *Zhong Ji* (CV 3), and *Gui Lai* (St 29). Choose 2-4 points from the above and moxa them directly with cones or over garlic, ginger, or Chinese onion.

I always prefer moxibustion method to needling for this condition and with good results.

2. Heavenly moxibustion: Mash 10 castor beans (Semen Ricini Communis [*Bi Ma Zi*]) into a paste and apply this to *Yong Quan* (Ki 1) on the side opposite to the welling abscess. This paste should be fixed in place with an adhesive plaster and changed 1 time each day.

Reference: There is a report of totally successful treatment of 204 cases of acute orchitis by moxibustion. The point *Yang Chi* (TB 4) alone was directly moxaed with 3 cones each treatment. One course consisted of 7 sessions. All the cases were cured within 1 course. The quickest cure was brought to pass in 10 hours. Sun Xue-quan: *Zhong Yi Za Zhi (J. of C.M.)* 1983; (4):8.

7
Intestinal Welling Abscess (Appendicitis)

The Golden Cabinet contains a passage describing intestinal welling abscess. It says:

> Intestinal welling abscess is a swelling glomus within the lower abdomen which is painful when pressed. It resembles dribbling urinary block but with normal urination. There is fever, spontaneous sweating, and aversion to cold from time to time. If the pulse is deep and slow, pus is not yet developed and one may use precipitation. Then blood should be precipitated. If the pulse is surging and rapid, pus has well developed and one can no longer use precipitation.

Besides *The Golden Cabinet*, a great many other classics also devote space to this disease. *The Mirror* is worth particular notice in this respect for it is the first Chinese classic to realize somewhat different locations of this disease in the abdomen. According to this work, intestinal *yong* is named large intestine welling abscess if it affects the area around the point *Tian Shu* (St 25). It is called small intestine *yong* if it affects the area around *Guan Yuan* (CV 4). It is called curling intestine welling abscess if it affects the umbilicus, and foot-contracting welling abscess if the right leg has to be contracted during the paroxysm.

Disease causes, disease mechanisms

As to the disease causes and progression of this disease, *The Origin* says,:

> Inordinate cold or heat and excessive joy or anger give evils a chance to interfere with the constructive and defensive. If they lodge in the intestines and meet with heat, the blood and qi will be heated and accumulate there, binding and gathering into welling abscess. This heat accumulates and does not disperse. Therefore, the blood and flesh decay, transforming into pus.

Cold and heat mean not only external cold and heat but cold and heat generated internally, for example, by eating too much cold or acrid food or drinks or fire transformed from depressed liver.

Treatment based on pattern discrimination

In regard to treatment, this disease is divided into two patterns:

1. Depression & stagnation pattern: This pattern is characterized by spasmodic abdominal pain which is worsened when the abdomen is pressed, abdominal distention and fullness, belching, torpid intake, nausea, retching and vomiting, normal defecation or constipation, and possibly slight aversion to cold and fever. The tongue is red with white or yellowish white fur, and the pulse is bowstring and tight.

Treatment principles: Move stasis and resolve stagnation, free the flow of the central qi. Select relevant points on the *yang ming* channel as the ruling points.

Formula: *Zhong Wan* (CV 12), *Da Heng* (Sp 15), *Lan Wei Xue* (M-LE-13), *Nei Ting* (St 44), *He Gu* (LI 4), and *Shang Ju Xu* (St 37)

Treatment method: Needle all these points using draining technique.

Explanation of the formula: *Lan Wei Xue* (M-LE-13) is a proven effective point for appendicitis. *Shang Ju Xu* (St 37) is at once a point on the stomach channel and the lower sea point of the large intestine. Combined with it, *He Gu* (LI 4) and *Zhong Wan* (CV 12) are able to clear heat from the intestines and stop pain. *Nei Ting* (St 44) frees the flow of the *yang ming* channel to resolve swelling, and *Da Heng* (Sp 15) is intended to fortify the spleen and supplement the central qi.

2. Accumulated heat pattern: This pattern is characterized by a mass in the right lower abdomen and long-lasting, intense pain in the abdomen which is tense and taut. This pain deters one from giving the abdomen the slightest touch. There is also nausea, retching and vomiting, constipation, short voidings of scant urine, and strong fever. The tongue is dark red with slimy, yellow fur, and the pulse is bowstring and rapid.

Treatment principles: Clear heat and disinhibit dampness, quicken the blood and transform stasis. Select relevant points on the *yang ming* and foot *tai yin* channel as the ruling ones.

Formula: *San Li* (St 36), *Da Chang Shu* (Bl 25), *Zhi Yang* (GV 9), *Fu Jie* (Sp 14), *Yin Ling Quan* (Sp 9), and *Lan Wei Xue* (M-LE-13)

Treatment method: Needle all these points using draining technique.

Other choice: Moxibustion: The frequently chosen points are on the *yang ming* channel, the controlling vessel, and the foot *jue yin* channel. Ruling points: *Lan Wei Xue* (M-LE-13), *Shang Ju Xu* (St 37), *Xue Hai* (Sp 10), *Da Dun* (Liv 1), and local *a shi* (tender) points. Auxiliary points: *Tian Shu* (St 25), *Qu Chi* (LI 11), *Wai Guan* (TB 5), *Zhou Jian* (M-UE-46), and *Da Chang Shu* (Bl 25).

Case history: A female, aged 20, complained of pain in her right lower abdomen with nausea and retching. The case was diagnosed as acute appendicitis. Needling was immediately performed at *Tian Shu* (St 25) bilaterally and the tender point a little distal to *San Li* (St 36) on the right leg. Two treatments and the condition was under control.

Reference: In a report on the electroacupuncture treatment of 40 cases of appendicitis, the ruling point selected was *Lan Wei Xue* (M-LE-13). The auxiliary points were *Tian Shu* (St 25) and *San Li* (St 36) on the right side. After strong stimulation was induced by hand, electrostimulation was done for 30 minutes. One treatment was given at intervals of 8-12 hours. Thirty cases were cured after 3-12 treatments; 4 showed marked improvement; and 6 were failures. Zhang Tian-hui: *Zhong Guo Zhen Jiu (Chin. Acu. & Mox.)* 1982; (3): 17.

Note: Acupuncture and moxibustion are effective for acute, simple appendicitis, and 2-3 treatments may send the patient to recovery. As to other types of this disease, however, acumoxatherapy can only be used as an auxiliary treatment.

General Index

A

A Concise Book 215
A Concise Formulary Book 2
A.D.V. Premaratue 116
abscesses (also see welling abscess and flat abscess)
abscesses, axillary welling 1, 48
abscesses, headless flat 55
abdominal distention 39, 86, 157, 176, 229, 233, 244
abdominal distention and pain exacerbated 39
abdominal pain 37-40, 86, 244
Academic Journal of Anhui C.M. Institute 104
aching 39, 40, 123, 145, 147, 171, 182, 184, 187, 188, 222
aching, generalized pain and 11
acne 21-23, 27, 37, 105, 113, 114, 119
acne rosacea 105
acne vulgaris 113
acupuncture, auricular 23
addictive papules 85, 88
allergic purpura 36, 37
alopecia 31, 123, 125
alopecia areata 123
American Journal of Acupuncture 116
An Aggrandisement to External Medicine 49
An Hui Zhong yi Xue Yuan Xue Bao 104
An Illustrated Supplement to the Classified 50
anal diseases 203
anal fissure 209
anaphylactic shock 127
anger and anxiety 225
angioma 215
animal bites 127
ankle sprain 23, 153-155
anus, splitting of the 209
appendicitis 5, 19, 233, 243-245
appetite, no 133
apprehensiveness 134
Artemisia Argyium 26
arthritis 55, 161, 187, 191, 193, 194
arthritis, rheumatic (osteoarthritis)187
arthritis, rheumatoid 193, 194
articular wind 187, 193
asthma 30
auricular acupuncture 23

B

Ba Du Gao 43
back sprain, upper 145
bedsores 25, 31, 103, 104
bee and wasp sting 127
belching 244
Ben Cao Cong Xin 26
bi (see impediment)
bladder damp heat pattern 40
bleeding, subcutaneous 39
blood, ejection of 39
body, cold 39, 40, 131, 175, 189
body, flaccid 157
boils, malign 57
bone fracture 23, 104
breast condition, fibrocystic 225
breast welling abscess 73-75
breath, bad 39
breath, shortness of 37, 39, 87, 130, 175, 222, 233
breathing, dyspneic difficult 39
breathing dyspneic with rales 130, 175
Bupleurum & Pueraria Decoction 66

C

Case Histories 49, 53, 56, 66, 69, 103, 122, 139, 208, 230
Causes 5, 6, 27, 28, 35, 36, 38, 41, 47, 48, 51, 52, 55, 57, 61, 63, 65, 69, 73, 79, 83, 85, 89, 93, 95, 101, 103, 105, 109, 113, 117, 121, 123, 133, 137, 143, 145, 147, 151, 153, 157, 161, 163, 167, 169, 171, 173, 179, 183, 187, 189, 193, 195, 201, 203, 207, 209, 211, 213, 215, 219, 221, 225, 233, 235, 239, 241, 243
central qi fall pattern 39
cervical fracture 140
cervical spondylosis 183, 186
Chai Hu Ge Gen Tang 66
channel & network vessel pattern discrimination 36
cheeks, bloated 65
cheeks, red 13, 37
Chen Ming 165
chest and rib-side pain 197
chest fullness and oppression 175
chest, pain and oppression in the 37
Chinese Acupuncture & Moxibustion 67, 71, 77, 81, 102, 111, 114, 116, 122, 144, 146, 149, 155, 165, 167, 170, 182, 186, 191, 195, 202, 205, 208, 218, 219, 224, 227, 245
Chinese Journal of Nursing 99
cinnabar toxins 61, 62
clove sores 10, 29, 57, 59
cold, aversion to 37, 39, 48, 61, 66, 125, 127, 130, 174, 175, 184, 187, 189, 201, 226, 243, 244
colds 25, 30
collapse, sudden 183
Collected Supplements to [the Theory of] 235
combination of channels of the same name 34
combination of exterior & interior 33
combination of front & back 33
combination of left & right 33

combination of local & distant points 32
combined needling & cupping 30
complexion of the affected skin, waxy, bright 173
conception, difficult 226
Concise Book 2, 215
constipation 11, 12, 35, 37-39, 48, 57, 75, 86, 89, 113, 114, 138, 207, 209, 229, 233, 244
corns 101
costal chondritis 197, 198
cough 30
coughing with scanty phlegm 37
coughing with thin phlegm 37
cupping 29, 30, 45, 48, 62, 70, 84, 86, 87, 90, 91, 94, 114, 118, 119, 127, 129, 134, 164, 165, 172, 181, 185, 189, 191, 195, 201, 207, 208, 222, 237
cupping, flash- 29
cupping, medicinal 30
cut, helping heal the 229
cutaneous neuritis 171, 172
cyst, ganglion 145, 146
cyst, sebaceous 219

D

Da Huo Luo Dan 155
Dan Xi Xin Fa 203
deafness 183
deformation impediment 193
dermatitis medicamentosa 37
dermatitis, seborrheic 37
dermatomyositis 37
dermatoses & infectious sores 35
Di Gu Pi Fen 80, 81, 104
diarrhea 39, 40, 86, 124, 138, 147, 207, 211, 216
Die Da Wan 155
digestion, swift, with rapid hungering 39
direction method 21
Dispel Rot Powder 229
Divinely Responding Classic 49, 59
dizziness 36-39, 123-125, 127, 130, 183-185, 223
dog bite, rabid 133, 135
Dong Tian Ao Zhi 129
draining & supplementing techniques 20
dreaming, profuse 36-39, 125, 183, 222, 225
drinks, desire for chilled 89
drooling from the mouth 134
dropsy 22

E

ears, ringing in the 39, 40, 123, 174, 183
ecchymosis 22, 36, 154
eczema 23, 27, 37, 83, 84, 211
eczema, chronic 37
eczema, perianal 211

elbow, taxed 167
electroacupuncture 23, 99, 154, 158, 164, 169, 170, 181, 185, 191, 199, 236, 239, 245
Emergency Formulas [to Keep] Behind the Elbow 1
Enlightening the Subtleties of External Medicine 127
Entering the Gate of Medicine 10
environmental excesses, six 5, 41, 137
ephidrosis 37
erysipelas 61
expulsion from within 15, 16
External Platform 2, 135
external treatment 15, 16
extremities, numbness in the 193
extremities, purple-colored, chilled 174, 175
eyes, dryness of the 38
eyes, red, swollen 38

F

face, fracture in the 138
face, swollen limbs and 37
facial complexion, chalky white 13
facial complexion, dull, somber 124, 174
facial complexion, pale 174, 231
facial complexion, red 38, 216
facial complexion, sallow yellow 36, 39, 176
facial complexion, somber white 39
facial complexion, somber white or sallow yellow 39
Fall & Knock Pills 155
fatigue 36, 37, 39, 80, 86, 87, 93, 125, 176, 193, 222, 223, 226
fever 11-13, 23, 32, 35, 40, 48, 51, 52, 55-57, 61, 66, 76, 127, 130, 134, 187-189, 241, 243, 244
fever and chills 12, 47, 56, 57, 65, 73, 75, 86
fever, low-grade 193
fever, slight 133
fever, tidal 13, 37, 189
fiber-severing 209
fibrocystic breast condition 225
fire girdle cinnabar 89
flaccid body 157
flat abscesses 1-3, 8, 51-53, 55, 57, 69
flat abscesses, headless 55
flat abscesses, sticking to the bone 55
food intake, low 39
food, no desire for 11, 12, 52, 66, 74, 233
Formulas Based on the Three Causes 137
Formulas [Worth a] Thousand [Pieces of] 2
Four Normalizations Clearing & Cooling Drink 66
fracture 23, 55, 104, 137-141
fracture, bone 23, 104
fracture, cervical 140
fracture in the face 138
fracture of the extremities 141
fracture, sternum & rib 140

Frankincense Paste 80
frostbite 24, 109-111
frozen sore 109
Fu Jian Zhong Yi Za Zhi 177
Fujian J. of C.M. 177
furuncles 10, 41

G

ganglion cyst 145, 146
gangrene 21
gastritis 30
Ge Hong 1
Generate Muscle [i.e., Flesh] Powder 122, 230
genitals, ulcerated 38
goiter 215-217
goiter, stone 215
Golden Cabinet Kidney Qi Pills 141
Great Compendium 19, 25

H

hair, dry, brittle 38
hands, numbness of the 183
He Nan Zhong Yi Za Zhi 59
head, clouded 11
head, prickly itching on, copious oily secretion 124
headache 11, 22, 48, 52, 61, 65, 73, 74, 88, 124, 133, 139, 183-185, 201, 241
Heart Attainment 47, 48
heart blood stasis pattern 38
heart palpitations 36, 37, 39, 87, 93, 123, 130, 183, 216, 223
heart yang vacuity pattern 37
heart yin vacuity pattern 37
heel pain 147, 148
hemafecia 37, 39, 95, 208
hematemesis 39
hematuria 37, 39
hemoptysis 39
hemorrhoids 2, 21, 22, 31, 33, 203, 204, 207-209, 240
herpes zoster 22, 37, 89, 91
hiccough 235-237
hives 22, 23, 35-37
hives, acute 37
hives, chronic 36, 37
hungering, swift digestion with rapid 39
hypertension 25
hypothermia 109, 111

I

Illustrated Supplement 50
Illustration of the Theories of External 51
Immortal Formula for Quickening Life 49, 53

impediment 30, 32, 161, 162, 169, 171, 173, 175, 179, 181, 183-185, 187-189, 193, 197
impediment, deformation 193
impediment, fixed 162, 171, 188
impediment, hot 188
impediment, migratory 161, 187
impediment, painful 162, 188
impediment, sinew 179, 181
impotence 40, 124, 125, 147, 159, 184
indigestion 30
Inner Classic 3, 7, 10, 16, 153, 161, 207, 215, 235
Inner Mongolia Journal of C..M. & Medicinals 102
insomnia 23, 36-39, 87, 93, 116, 123-125, 183, 185, 216, 222, 225
internal damage 6
intestinal gripping pain 23
intestinal welling abscess 5, 243
irritability 96, 139, 225
itching 11, 19, 22, 27, 38, 42, 51, 52, 57, 58, 79, 83-85, 88, 94, 105, 106, 117, 118, 121-125, 127, 133, 173, 208, 211
itching on the head with copious oily secretion, prickly 124

J, K

Journal of Integrated Chinese & Western Medicine 77
jaundice 38
Jiang Guan 53
Jiang Su Zhong Yi Za Zhi 91
Jiangsu Journal of C.M. 91
Jie Du Zi Jin Gao 80
Jin Gui Shen Qi Wan 104, 141
Jin Gui Yi 143
Jing Yue Quan Shu 47, 239
Jing-yue's Complete Book 239
joint deformation 193
Journal of Chinese Medicine 44
kidney stones 23
kidney yang vacuity pattern 40
kidney yin vacuity pattern 39

L

large intestine damp heat pattern 37
Lei Jing Tu Yi 50
lesions, dark purple 113
lesions, red with nodular papules 113
lesions, soft tissue 23
Li Dong-yuan 3
Li Feng 102, 114
Li Yan 10
limbs, chilled 147, 174, 226
limbs, heavy, numb 183
limbs, numbness of the 38

limbs, swollen 37, 39, 40
Ling Shu 1, 7
lips, purplish 174
listlessness 39, 52
Liu Juan Zi Gui Yi Fang 2
liver blood vacuity pattern 38
liver channel cold dampness pattern 38
liver fire pattern, effulgent 38
liver qi depression & binding pattern 38
liver-gallbladder damp heat pattern 38
low back and knees, aching and flaccid 40
low back, aching 40, 222
low back pain 40, 125, 143, 148
low back soreness 174
low back, wrenching of the 143, 145
lower abdominal pain 38
Lu Lin 53
lumbar sprain, acute 143
lung channel heat pattern 37
lung qi vacuity pattern 37
lung yin vacuity pattern 37
Luo Yan 186
lupus erythmatosus 37
Lycium Root Bark Powder 80, 81, 104
lymphadenopathy 22, 26

M

Ma Pei Zhi Wai Ke Yi An 69
Major Quicken the Network Vessels Elixir 155
mammary fibroadenoma 221
mammary node 221, 225
mandibular pain 199
mastitis, acute 73, 77
measles 37, 55
melancholy 225
memory, impaired 37, 123
menstrual flow, profuse 39
menstrual irregularity 38, 85, 87, 124, 138, 174, 222, 224, 225
menstruation, painful 38, 87
miliaria 42
Ming Yi Lei An 53
miscarriage, liability to 226
mouth, a bitter taste in the 38, 56, 89, 91, 216
mouth, drooling from the 134
mouth, dry, but no desire to drink 174
mouth ulcers 38
move, disinclination to 39
moxa cones 26, 27
moxa roll 25, 28, 70, 75, 90, 110, 151, 176, 191, 200, 202, 204, 207, 236
moxibustion, flash- 28
moxibustion, heavenly 28, 242
moxibustion, indirect 27, 43

Moxibustion Methods for Welling & Flat Abscesses 3
moxibustion, methods of 25, 26
moxibustion, non-scarring 27
Moxibustion, Riding the Bamboo Horse 3
moxibustion, scarring 26, 27
mumps 65, 67
myotenositis musculi supraspinati 179, 180

N

neck and shoulder pain 183
neck, crick in the 201
neck, stiffness and pain in the 183
neck welling abscess 47
needle, cutaneous 22, 106, 114, 125, 127, 144, 171, 176, 179, 208, 217, 240
needle, three-edged 22, 30, 114, 180, 207
needle, water 24
needling, cluster 22
needling, dispersed 22
needling, distant selection 31, 32
needling, fire- 21, 56, 76, 91, 97, 99, 102, 114, 121, 122, 146, 165, 204, 208
needling, lifting & thrusting method 21
needling, local selection 31
needling methods 19
needling, opening & shutting method 21
needling, point selection 3, 23, 31, 32, 167
needling, proximate selection 31
needling techniques for hastening the qi 20
needling the network vessels 22
needling, tip 22
needling, twirling method 21
needling, varying the speed method 21
Nei Jing 3
Nei Mong Zhong Yi Yao Za Zhi 102
neuralgia, post-herpetic 90
neuritis, cutaneous 171, 172
neurodermatitis 22, 36, 93, 94
Newly Collated Materia Medica 26
night sweats 13, 37, 39, 189
nodulations 36, 41, 42, 44, 222, 223
nodulations, mole cricket 42, 44
nodulations, summerheat 42
nodules, subcutaneous 36
Norms 41, 95
nosebleed 39
numbness 19, 22, 36, 38, 161, 171, 172, 183-185, 193, 229
numbness in the extremities 193
numbness of the hands 183
numbness of the limbs 38

O

oral cavity, ulceration of the 37
orchitis, acute 241, 242
Orthodox Gathering 16, 17, 27, 59, 65, 66, 73, 80, 83, 95, 123, 129, 133, 219
Orthodox Gathering of External Medicine 16
orthopedics 137, 148
osteomyelitis, pyogenic 55
oxhide lichen 93

P

papules, addictive 85, 88
paraplegia, traumatic 157, 160
pattern discrimination, channel & network vessel 36
penis, pain in the 40
periarthritis of the shoulder 163
phlebitis 22
piriformis syndrome 195
Pithy Essentials of External Medicine 237
Pivotal Essentials of External Medicine 17, 221
point selection 3, 23, 31, 32, 167
points, ruling & auxiliary 32
pricking powder 113
Prolong Life by Protecting the Origin 27, 63
pruritus 35, 37
psoriasis 23, 30, 36, 117, 119
purpura, allergic 36, 37
pus 7, 10-12, 15, 17, 21, 26, 29, 41, 44, 48, 49, 51, 52, 55-59, 66, 73, 76, 80, 90, 95, 121, 122, 214, 243
pyogenic infection 57
pyogenic osteomyelitis 55

Q

qi & blood pattern discrimination 36
qi, forked 145
qi goiter 215-217
qi, obtaining the 19, 21, 154
Qi Zhu Ma Jiu Fa 3
Qian Jin Fang 2
Qian Jin Yi Fang 2
Qu Fu San 229, 230

R

raving 8, 11, 58, 130, 131
rectum, prolapse of the 39, 203-205
Resolve Toxins Purple Gold Paste 80
respiration method 21
rheumatic arthritis 187
rheumatoid arthritis 193, 194
rhomboideus strain 181, 182

rib-side pain 38, 58, 140, 197, 216, 225, 233
ringworm 22, 27
Ru Xiang Gao 80
Ru Yi Jin Huang San 66
Rules & Laws Within the Gate of Medicine 6

S

Sagelike Formulas 26, 41
San Xiang Gao 80
San Yin Fang 137
San Yin Ji Yi Bing Zheng Fang Lun 5
scalp, wind glossy 123
sciatica 169, 170
scleroderma 37, 173, 176, 177
scleroderma, systemic 173
scrofula 1, 21, 27, 64
scrofulous lumps 63, 64
scrotum, contraction of the 38
sebaceous cyst 219
Secret Essentials of the External Platform 2
Secret Records of External Medicine 7
seminal emission 39, 40, 124, 125, 138, 174
septicemia 58
sexual desire, reduced 226
Shan Dong Zhong Yi Za Zhi 144
Shan Xi Zhong Yi Za Zhi 62, 119, 135
Shang Hai Zhen Jiu Za Zhi 91, 98, 172, 176
Shang Hai Zhong Yi Yao Za Zhi 94
Shanghai J. of Acu. & Mox. 91, 98, 172, 176
Shanghai J. of C.M. 94
shank sore 79
Shanxi J. of C.M. 119
Shen Nong Ben Cao Jing 215
Shen Ying Jing 49
Sheng Ji San 64, 79, 122, 230
Sheng Ji Zong Lu 61
Shi Quan Da Bu Wan 104
shivering, cold 11
shoulder, periarthritis of the 163
shoulder wind, exposed 163-165, 169, 179
Shou Shi Bao Yuan 27, 63
Si Chuan Zhong Yi 97, 172
Si Shun Qing Liang Yin 66
Sichuan C.M. 97
Simple Questions 1, 57, 58, 113, 135, 157, 203
sinew binding 145
sinew goiter 215
sinew impediment 179, 181
sinews, damaged 153, 154
sinews, hypertonicity of the 133
sitting wind 211
skin, dryness of the 38
skin impediment 171, 173, 175
skin, waxy, bright complexion of the affected 173

skull fracture 139
sleep, poor 124
sloughing flat abscesses 69
small intestine damp heat pattern 38
snake bite 29, 129
snake cinnabar 89
snake girdle 89
soft tissue lesions 23
spasm and tremors arising on drinking 134
speak, disinclination to 225, 231
spirit abstraction 37, 104
spirit, clouded 8, 11, 58, 65, 130, 131, 138
spleen qi vacuity pattern 39
sprain 22, 23, 143, 145, 153-155, 181
sternum & rib fracture 140
stomach & intestines damp heat pattern 39
stools, blood in the 37
stools, loose 124, 174, 176, 226
Su Wen 1
Supplement 2, 16-18, 20, 44, 50, 52, 53, 55, 56, 70, 80, 87, 88, 94, 98, 103, 124, 135, 138, 140, 143, 147, 158, 159, 174, 204, 223, 226, 236, 239, 244
sweating, copious spontaneous 134
sweating, profuse 216
sweating, spontaneous 13, 35-37, 134, 223, 243
sweats, night 13, 37, 39, 189

T

Tai Ping Sheng Hui Fang 2, 26
tail bone pain 151
temporomandibular joint syndrome 199
tennis elbow 31, 167
The Classified Case Histories from 53
The Essence & Essentials of External 8
The Great Collection for External 12
The Great Compendium of Acupuncture 19
The Heart Attainment of External Medicine 47
The Mirror 73, 101, 105, 109, 113, 203, 243
The Norms 41, 95
The Norms of Patterns & their Treatment 41
The Occult Purport of Heaven [Observed] 129
The Origins 2, 41, 51, 85, 109, 153
The Spiritual Pivot 1, 7, 19, 25, 55, 69, 157, 158, 161
The Supplement to the Formulas [Worth] 2
The Treatise on Diseases, their Symptoms 5
thin, white phlegm 175
thirst 12, 35, 37-39, 41, 47, 51, 57, 74, 75, 105, 117, 134, 188, 189, 235
thirst and a desire for cold drinks 39
thirst and a desire for water 38, 105
Thousand Pieces of Gold 2
Three Fragrances Paste 80
throat, constriction of the 133
throat, dry 39, 89

thromboangitis obliterans 69, 70
thyroid adenoma 215, 218
thyroid adenoma, simple diffuse 215
thyroid carcinoma 215
tongue and mouth, dry 40
torpid intake 39, 74, 83, 86, 87, 124, 176, 193, 216, 223, 226, 244
torticollis 201
toxins 6-11, 15, 17-22, 29, 32, 36, 42-44, 48, 49, 51, 52, 56-59, 61, 62, 65, 66, 70, 73, 76, 79, 80, 83, 89, 90, 98, 99, 106, 107, 109, 114, 127, 129-131, 133-135, 203, 214, 225, 241
traumatic accidents 6
traumatic paraplegia 157, 160
traumatology 137, 148
Treatise on the Origins & Symptoms of 2
treatment, external 15, 16
tumors 213

U

ulceration 26, 30, 37, 79, 80, 104, 122
ulceration of the oral cavity 37
urinary block 135, 229, 239, 243
urinary incontinence 139, 141, 157, 183
urinary retention 239, 240
urinary urgency 40
urine, frequent voiding of 40
urine, long voidings of clear 174
urine, reddish 38, 39
urine, short voidings of scanty 38, 89, 105
urticaria 85, 88

V

varicosities 22
varicosity syndrome 79
vexation 6, 11, 37, 38, 58, 74, 84, 86, 89, 94, 113, 117, 130, 134, 188, 189, 216, 221, 222, 225
viscera & bowel pattern discrimination 37
vision, blurred 130
vision, impaired 183
vitamin B 205
vitiligo 23, 27, 115, 116
voice, weak 37

W

Wai Ke Fa Hui 49
Wai Ke Jing Yao 8, 237
Wai Ke Jiu Fa Lun Cui Xin Shu 3
Wai Ke Li Li 51
Wai Ke Mi Lu 7
Wai Ke Qi Xuan 8, 127
Wai Ke Quan Sheng Ji 69

Wai Ke Zheng Zhi Quan Shu 73
Wai Ke Zheng Zong 16
Wai Tai Mi Yao 2
Wang Bin 113
Wang Ji 51, 194
Wang Tao 2
warts 21, 95-99
warts, flat 96
warts, plantar 95, 99
water needle 24
weakness, generalized 37, 80
weight loss 193
welling abscesses, axillary 1, 48
welling abscess, external kidney 241
welling abscess, intestinal 5, 243
welling abscess, neck 47
wet foot qi 121
white patch has distinct boundaries 115
white patch has no distinct boundaries 115
white patch wind 115, 116
white sore 117
wilting 24, 158, 169, 183, 184, 193
wind damp impediment pain 30
wind dampness disease 187
wind, jumping round 169
wrist sprain 153

X, Y

Xian Fang Huo Ming Yin 49, 53, 70
Xiao Pin Fang 2
Xu Ming Yi Lei An 53
Xue Ji 8, 17, 49, 221
Yang Yi Da Quan 12
Yi Men Fa Lu 6
Yi Xue Ru Men 10
Yi Zheng Gu Shang Ke Za Zhi 148
Yong Ju Jiu Fa 3

Z

Zhang Zi-he 3
Zhao Dong 97
Zhe Jiang Zhong Yi Za Zhi 44, 119, 177, 194, 200
Zhen Jiu Da Cheng 19
Zhen Jiu Zi Sheng Jing 88
Zheng Zhi Hui Bu 235
Zheng Zhi Yao Jue 203
Zheng Zhi Zhun Sheng 41
Zhong Guo Zhen Jiu 53, 67, 71, 77, 81, 102, 111, 114, 116, 122, 144, 146, 149, 155, 165, 167, 170, 182, 186, 191, 195, 202, 205, 208, 218, 219, 224, 227, 245
Zhong guo Zhong 148
Zhong Hua Hu Li Xue Za Zhi 99
Zhong Xi Yi Jie He Za Zhi 77
Zhong Yi Za Zhi 44, 53, 59, 62, 91, 111, 119, 135, 144, 177, 194, 200, 242
Zhou Hou Bei Ji Fang 1
Zhu Bing Yuan Hou Lun 2

OTHER BOOKS ON CHINESE MEDICINE AVAILABLE FROM BLUE POPPY PRESS
1775 Linden Ave ○ Boulder, CO 80304
For ordering 1-800-487-9296
PH. 303\447-8372 FAX 303\447-0740 email 102151.1614@compuserve.com

A COMPENDIUM OF TCM PATTERNS & TREATMENTS by Bob Flaws & Daniel Finney, ISBN 0-936185-70-8, $29.95

A HANDBOOK of TCM PEDIATRICS by Bob Flaws, ISBN 0-936185-72-4, $49.95

A HANDBOOK OF TRADITIONAL CHINESE DERMATOLOGY by Liang Jian-hui, trans. by Zhang Ting-liang & Bob Flaws, ISBN 0-936185-07-4 $17.95

A HANDBOOK OF TRADITIONAL CHINESE GYNECOLOGY by Zhejiang College of TCM, trans. by Zhang Ting-liang, ISBN 0-936185-06-6 (2nd edit.) $21.95

A HANDBOOK OF TCM UROLOGY & MALE SEXUAL DYSFUNCTION by Anna Lin, OMD, ISBN 0-936185-36-8, $16.95

A NEW AMERICAN ACUPUNCTURE: Acupuncture Osteopathy, by Mark Seem, ISBN 0-936185-44-9, $22.95

ACUPUNCTURE AND MOXIBUSTION FORMULAS & TREATMENTS by Cheng Dan-an, trans. by Wu Ming, ISBN 0-936185-68-6, $22.95

ACUTE ABDOMINAL SYNDROMES: Their Diagnosis & Treatment by Combined Chinese-Western Medicine by Alon Marcus, ISBN 0-936185-31-7 $16.95

AGING & BLOOD STASIS: A New TCM Approach to Geriatrics by Yan De-Xin, ISBN 0-936185-63-5, $21.95

AIDS & ITS TREATMENT ACCORDING TO TRADITIONAL CHINESE MEDICINE by Huang Bing-shan, trans. by Fu-Di & Bob Flaws, ISBN 0-936185-28-7 $25.95

ARISAL OF THE CLEAR: A Simple Guide to Healthy Eating According to Traditional Chinese Medicine by Bob Flaws, ISBN #-936185-27-9 $10.95

CHINESE MEDICAL PALMISTRY: Your Health in Your Hand, by Zong Xiao-fan & Gary Liscum, ISBN 0-936185-64-3, $15.95

CHINESE MEDICINAL TEAS: Simple, Proven, Folk Formulas for Common Diseases & Promoting Health, by Zong Xiao-fan & Gary Liscum, ISBN 0-936185-76-7, $19.95

CHINESE MEDICINAL WINES & ELIXIRS by Bob Flaws, ISBN 0-936185-58-9, $18.95

CHINESE PEDIATRIC MASSAGE THERAPY A Parent's & Practitioner's Guide to the Treatment and Prevention of Childhood Disease, by Fan Ya-li. ISBN 0-936185-54-6, $12.95

CHINESE SELF-MASSAGE: The Easy Way to Health; by Fan Ya-li, ISBN 0-936185-74-0, $15.95

CLASSICAL MOXIBUSTION SKILLS IN CONTEMPORARY CLINICAL PRACTICE by Sung Baek, ISBN 0-936185-16-3 $12.95

ENDOMETRIOSIS & INFERTILITY AND TCM: A Laywoman's Guide by Bob Flaws ISBN 0-936185-14-7 $10.95

EXTRA TREATISES BASED ON INVESTIGATION & INQUIRY: A Translation of Zhu Dan-xi's *Ge Zhi Yu Lun*, trans. by Yang Shou-zhong & Duan Wu-jin, ISBN 0-936185-53-8, $15.95

FIRE IN THE VALLEY: The TCM Diagnosis and Treatment of Vaginal Diseases by Bob Flaws ISBN 0-936185-25-2 $18.95

FLESHING OUT THE BONES: The Importance of Case Histories in Chinese Medicine by Charles Chace. ISBN 0-936185-30-9, $18.95

FU QING-ZHU'S GYNECOLOGY trans. by Yang Shou-zhong and Liu Da-wei, ISBN 0-936185-35-X, $22.95

FULFILLING THE ESSENCE: A Handbook of Traditional & Contemporary Chinese Treatments for Female Infertility by Bob Flaws. ISBN 0-936185-48-1, $19.95

HIGHLIGHTS OF ANCIENT ACUPUNCTURE PRESCRIPTIONS trans. by Honora Lee Wolfe & Rose Crescenz ISBN 0-936185-23-6 $14.95

How to Have a **HEALTHY PREGNANCY, HEALTHY BIRTH** with Traditional Chinese Medicine by Honora Lee Wolfe, ISBN 0-936185-40-6, $9.95

HOW TO WRITE A TCM HERBAL FORMULA A Logical Methodology for the Formulation & Administration of Chinese Herbal Medicine in Decoction, by Bob Flaws, ISBN 0-936185-49-X, $10.95

IMPERIAL SECRETS OF HEALTH & LONGEVITY by Bob Flaws, ISBN 0-936185-51-1, $9.95

KEEPING YOUR CHILD HEALTHY WITH CHINESE MEDICINE by Bob Flaws, ISBN 0-936185-71-6, $15.95

Li Dong-yuan's **TREATISE ON THE SPLEEN & STOMACH**, A Translation of the *Pi Wei Lun* by Yang Shou-zhong & Li Jian-yong, ISBN 0-936185-41-4, $22.95

LOW BACK PAIN: Care & Prevention with Traditional Chinese Medicine by Douglas Frank, ISBN 0-936185-66-X, $9.95

MASTER HUA'S CLASSIC OF THE CENTRAL VISCERA by Hua Tuo, translated by Yang Shou-zhong, ISBN 0-936185-43-0, $21.95

MASTER TONG'S ACUPUNCTURE: An Ancient Lineage for Modern Practice, trans. and commentary by Miriam Lee, OMD, ISBN 0-936185-37-6, $19.95

MENOPAUSE, A Second Spring: Making A Smooth Transition with Traditional Chinese Medicine by Honora Wolfe ISBN 0-936185-18-X, 4th edition, $14.95

MIGRAINES & TRADITIONAL CHINESE MEDICINE: A Layperson's Guide by Bob Flaws ISBN 0-936185-15-5 $11.95

PAO ZHI: An Introduction to the Use of Processed Chinese Medicinals to Enhance Therapeutic Effects by Philippe Sionneau, translated by Bob Flaws, ISBN 0-936185-62-7, $34.95

PATH OF PREGNANCY, VOL. II, Postpartum Diseases by Bob Flaws, ISBN 0-936185-42-2, $19.95

PATH OF PREGNANCY, VOL. I, Gestational Disorders by Bob Flaws, ISBN 0-936185-39-2, $19.95

PEDIATRIC BRONCHITIS: ITS CAUSE, DIAGNOSIS & TREATMENT ACCORDING TO TRADITIONAL CHINESE MEDICINE trans. by Gao Yu-li and Bob Flaws, ISBN 0-936185-26-0 $15.95

PRINCE WEN HUI'S COOK: Chinese Dietary Therapy by Bob Flaws & Honora Lee Wolfe, ISBN 0-912111-05-4, $12.95 (Published by Paradigm Press, Brookline, MA)

RECENT TCM RESEARCH FROM CHINA trans. by Bob Flaws & Charles Chace. ISBN 0-936185-56-2, $18.95

SCATOLOGY & THE GATE OF LIFE: The Role of the Large Intestine in Immunity, An Integrated Chinese-Western Approach by Bob Flaws ISBN 0-936185-20-1 $16.95

SECRET SHAOLIN FORMULAS FOR THE TREATMENT OF EXTERNAL INJURY by De Qian, translated by Zhang Ting-liang and Bob Flaws, ISBN 0-936185-08-2, $18.95

SEVENTY ESSENTIAL TCM FORMULAS FOR BEGINNERS by Bob Flaws, ISBN 0-936185-59-7, $19.95

STATEMENTS OF FACT IN TRADITIONAL CHINESE MEDICINE by Bob Flaws. ISBN 0-936185-52-X, $12.95

STICKING TO THE POINT: A Rational Methodology for the Step by Step Administration of an Acupuncture Treatment by Bob Flaws ISBN 0-936185-17-1 $17.95

THE BOOK OF JOOK: Chinese Medicinal Porridges, A Healthy Alternative to the Typical Western Breakfast by Bob Flaws, ISBN 0-936185-60-0, $16.95

THE BREAST CONNECTION: A Laywoman's Guide to the Treatment of Breast Disease by Chinese Medicine by Honora Lee Wolfe ISBN 0-936185-13-9 $10.95

THE DAO OF INCREASING LONGEVITY AND CONSERVING ONE'S LIFE by Anna Lin & Bob Flaws, ISBN 0-936185-24-4 $18.95

THE DIVINELY RESPONDING CLASSIC: A Translation of the *Shen Ying Jing* from the *Zhen Jiu Da Cheng* by Yang Shou-zhong & Liu Feng-ting, ISBN 0-936185-55-4, $18.95

THE HEART & ESSENCE Of Dan-xi's Methods of Treatment by Zhu Dan-xi, trans. by Yang Shou-zhong. ISBN 0-936185-50-3, $24.95

THE MEDICAL I CHING: Oracle of the Healer Within by Miki Shima, ISBN 0-936185-38-4, $19.95

THE PULSE CLASSIC: A Translation of the *Mai Jing* by Yang Shou-zhong ISBN 0-936185-75-9, $54.95

THE SECRET OF CHINESE PULSE DIAGNOSIS by Bob Flaws, ISBN 0-936185-67-8, $17.95

THE SYSTEMATIC CLASSIC OF ACUPUNCTURE & MOXIBUSTION by Huang-fu Mi, trans. by Yang Shou-zhong and Charles Chace, ISBN 0-936185-29-5, hardback edition, $79.95

THE TREATMENT OF DISEASE IN TCM, Vol I: Diseases of the Head & Face Including Mental/Emotional Disorders by Philippe Sionneau & Lü Gang, ISBN 0-936185-69-4, $21.95

THE TREATMENT OF DISEASE IN TCM, Vol. II: Diseases of the Eyes, Ears, Nose, & Throat by Philippe Sionneau & Lü Gang, ISBN 0-936185-69-4, $21.95

THE TREATMENT OF DISEASE IN TCM, Vol. III: Diseases of the Mouth, Lips, Tongue, Teeth, & Gums by Philippe Sionneau, ISBN 0-936185-79-1, $21.95